PREVENTION OF FOOTBALL INJURIES

PREVENTION OF

Protecting the Health
of the Student Athlete

FOOTBALL INJURIES

O. CHARLES OLSON, M.D.

Spokane, Washington

LEA & FEBIGER Philadelphia, 1971

Health Education,
Physical Education, and
Recreation Series

RUTH ABERNATHY, Ph.D., EDITORIAL ADVISER
Director, School of Physical and Health Education,
University of Washington, Seattle, Washington, 98105

RC 1220
. F6 Ø47

ISBN 0-8121-0346-7
Library of Congress Catalog Card Number 70–157472
Printed in the United States of America

To Mark, Craig, and Eric whose interest and participation in competitive sports aroused their Dad's curiosity and interest in the field of sports medicine and related health problems.

FOREWORD

EVERY person in coaching today should have a sound understanding of sports medicine and a working knowledge of the most current thinking of doctors relative to sports-associated injuries and disabilities. From the time I started coaching 42 years ago, tremendous strides have been made in the field of sports medicine. We know so much more today about the cause and treatment of athletic injuries that it becomes an inescapable responsibility for every coach, every team physician, and every trainer to keep himself informed on the most recent advances in this area of medicine. While no coach should pretend either to diagnose or to administer treatment, he should know enough to take the maximum precautions for his players to avoid injuries.

Dr. O. Charles Olson has made a contribution to the field of sports medicine with the publication of this book. The fact that three of his sons were fine athletes has no doubt deepened his interest in this particular field of inquiry and, as a result, has offered all those involved with athletics a chance to gain some insights and a body of practical knowledge about the health of the athlete.

I think this book will have a particular impact for high school athletics. Dr. Olson's statement that a team physician "enters a different world of medicine" is certainly true. The language of the coach and the athlete in the locker room is different than that of his office patients. The pseudo-scientific medical terms used by the coach, such as "hip pointer," are an entirely new language for the team physician. It is important that team physicians be familiar with the special vocabulary of coaching.

Dr. Olson writes with the layman in mind to such an extent that it is not necessary to have a medical degree to understand it. At the same time, the book is technically detailed enough to be meaningful to physicians.

Dr. Olson deals with the realities of today's coaching in the context of procedures of play and the resulting implications of these practices relative to athletic medicine.

For example, he deals with the technique of tackling in football commonly known as "spearing." This means hitting the opponent with the head. One study of high school players indicated that 60% of the head injuries and 44% of neck injuries came from this practice. His conclusion: spearing must not be taught and, further, must be outlawed. In addition, Dr. Olson says the player must be coached to strike the opponent with his head up, thus keeping the proper flex on the neck.

This is a sample of the kind of practical medical advice available to the coach. In other sections of the book he addresses himself to physicians and trainers; for example, what they should know about strength loss and necessary recovery time after exercising to fatigue.

Dr. Olson's book is a valuable contribution to the field of athletics in general and sports medicine in particular.

LEN CASANOVA

PREFACE

THE material in this book is basically a presentation of the major principles to be learned and practiced in the *prevention* of football injuries and in safeguarding the health of the players.

The contents are directed mainly to the high school team physicians and the high school coaches and trainers who may have some basic knowledge of injury prevention and general health care but would like more specifics.

Most colleges and universities learned long ago that a knowledgeable, motivated, and enthusiastic team physician is a most important member of the athletic department and that his supervision and responsibility in safeguarding the health of the athlete are of prime importance. There is no reason to believe that the team physician at the high school level should play any less important a role, and indeed may even play a more important one in indoctrinating players, coaches, and trainers in the fundamental aspects of health care and injury prevention in this younger age group.

It is my intention that this book will serve as a manual and guide for setting up a comprehensive program of adequate medical care and injury prevention in schools where such a program does not presently exist. Perhaps some of the ideas contained in this book will serve to improve already existing programs as well. The book does not deal with the treatment of football injuries. Many fine books have been published on this subject (see Appendix).

There may be some statements in this book that are open to discussion and perhaps not all readers will fully agree. I have not assumed that this is the "last word" but feel it is at least a "first word" in emphasizing the major areas of injury prevention and health care for the football player.

I am in the private practice of internal medicine and developed my interest in the medical aspects of sports about a dozen years ago when my three sons began participating in competitive athletics, starting in grade school and high school and continuing for two of them into major college athletics. There is probably no greater stimulus to a physician's interest in sports medicine than having members of his family participating and perhaps there likewise is no greater pleasure and thrill.

From my own personal interest and participation as a team physician, I was able to stimulate our county medical society to organize a Committee on the Medical Aspects of Sports and thus to start an adequate and comprehensive program for medical supervision and care of the athletes in all the high schools in our community. This program has continued and expanded and is rending an important and vital service to the individual athlete, to the schools, and to the community.

The point I wish to make is that it takes only one or two motivated physicians to "get the show on the road" and provide the medical help that is so badly needed. A recent survey showed that almost half of the high schools in the United States do not have appointed physicians supervising health care and injury prevention. Certainly every high school in this country that participates in competitive athletics is entitled to a team physician. I firmly believe that physicians can and should make a greater effort in this aspect of community service.

O. CHARLES OLSON

Spokane, Washington

ACKNOWLEDGMENTS

MANY people have given me help in preparing this book. I am grateful to many team physicians, trainers, and coaches throughout the country who have shared their knowledge, experience and ideas. I am particularly grateful to Robert L. Bartlett, an outstanding high school coach from 1940 to 1964 and with whom I served as team physician for 7 years at Lewis and Clark High School in Spokane, Washington, for his technical assistance. I also wish to thank Mr. Dick Vandervoort, Head Trainer for Washington State University Athletic Department, for his assistance in the preparation of the chapter on protective equipment. I am equally grateful to Dr. Otto O. Stevens for his suggestions concerning mouth protectors. Dr. Stevens has done outstanding work with our high school athletes in evaluating mouth protectors and recently wrote the chapter on Prevention of Oral Injuries in Athletes for the book entitled, *Traumatic Dental Injuries*.

I wish to thank Dr. Jack Watkins, an outstanding orthopedic surgeon, for his suggestions and recommendations.

My dietitian, Mrs. Roberta Omans, has not only helped in the preparation of the dietary instructions in this book, but has spent many hours typing and retyping the manuscript, for which I am grateful.

I feel deeply honored to have my good friend Mr. Len Casanova write the Foreword to this book. Len Casanova, known to most of the athletic fraternity as "Cas," has devoted his life work to young athletes and has been aptly described as a man who has "molded hearts and minds, as well as bodies." Cas has enjoyed an outstanding career in coaching football, beginning in 1928 as a high school coach and progressing on to Santa Clara, Pittsburgh, and Oregon, followed by four years as Athletic Director at the University of Oregon. We wish him well in his new position as Associate Director of University Relations.

Last but not least, I am very grateful to all the athletes I have had the pleasure and privilege of working for and with—they have contributed in a great measure to this book.

O.C.O.

CONTENTS

Chapter 1

INTRODUCTION

Football is properly described as a contact sport but it can equally be described as a collision sport. I must remind you of the formula most of us learned in high school physics—$E = \frac{1}{2}M \times V^2$, in which E is the energy expended, M is mass or weight, and V is the velocity. We could conclude from this that the bigger athlete who moves faster must create more energy and thus hit harder —and in doing so may inflict or sustain injury in this delivery of energy.

With more skillful coaching of improved athletes, the game of football has become faster and tougher and thus the incidence of *some* injuries has increased, as would be expected. However, the incidence of other types of injury has decreased. It is the ultimate aim of all persons interested in the game to *decrease* the incidence of all types of injuries. If all physicians, coaches, trainers, and parents will take more time and effort to teach the players the fundamentals of injury prevention, then I am sure the incidence of all injuries will decrease and the severity of others will be less.

Statistics on high school football injuries are valuable for two reasons—they enable us to analyze and evaluate and thus take proper steps to try to prevent similar injuries in the future, and they furnish information as to the trends in both numbers and types of injuries. I am grateful to Mr. Clifford B. Fagan, Executive Secretary for the National Federation of State High School Athletic Associations for furnishing me with the latest statistics on high school football injuries and fatalities.

At the present time about 900,000 high school boys are playing interscholastic football in the United States. How many of these boys sustain a reportable injury per season? On a national basis, about 19 boys per 100 sustain such an injury. This does not infer that these are major injuries and no figures are presently available on a national basis to define exactly what type of injury occurred. Many injuries are not reported. What constitutes a significant injury is another variable factor, thus it is a difficult matter to report valid and reliable figures on a national scale.

Direct football fatalities in high school players averaged 15.66 per year over the past 12 years for a total of 190 deaths. The yearly fatality rate has been slightly higher in the past 4 years than the 12 year average, namely 20 in 1969; 26 in 1968; 17 in 1967; 21 in 1966. However, this is due, at least in part, to the greater number of participants as well as the greater number of games played. Many high schools now field a Freshman team as well as a Junior Varsity team in interscholastic competition, whereas a few years ago they probably only competed on the varsity basis.

The average age for fatal injury was 16 years and the incidence was 1.82 per 100,000 participants. Defined in man-hours of exposure, there were approximately 143,000,000 man-hours of exposure and thus one death in 7,150,000 hours of exposure. Football is actually not a high-risk activity as regards fatal injuries. Nine times as many young men die in automobile accidents per man-hour of exposure as die on the football field. It seems obvious that the football field is a far safer place than the high-speed highways.

There are three basic and fundamental considerations that seem most important in any discussion of prevention of athletic injuries.

The first and probably the most important is the *selection of the coach*. The head coach is undoubtedly the number one man in the prevention of injuries. A good coach has many responsibilities and he must be emotionally stable, morally sound, and an excellent teacher and leader. The coach must be a disciple of thorough and proper conditioning and must teach the athletes the technique of individual and team play as well as proper and skillful coordination. The coach selects adequate protective equipment and fits it to each player and teaches him how to wear it properly. The coach must always be thinking in terms of *safety to the players* which would include discouraging tactics that may increase the hazards and the incidence of injuries; carefully analyzing injuries that do occur in order to determine what caused them and how to avoid them in the future; and carrying out carefully planned practice sessions of reasonable duration to avoid injuries that so often occur in the tired athlete. The coach and the team always want to play to win but the desire to win must never be so great as to contribute to injuries of the players.

Any high school coach who has more than one or two players disabled by injuries in the first 3 weeks of practice is neglecting one or more of the fundamental aspects of injury prevention, and most frequently this is due either to too early contact practice in a poorly conditioned player or to ignorance or neglect of proper techniques.

The second and equally important consideration is good medical care or utilizing the popular term—*safeguarding the health of the athlete*. At the high school level this is primarily the responsibility of the team physician with some help from the student trainer—at the college level the graduate trainer is a most important member of the medical team. The team physician's decisions in matters of injuries and health care must be absolute and unquestioned.

The third consideration in the prevention of injuries is *good equipment*, properly selected, properly worn, and kept in good repair.

In the following chapters I have written in some detail on all the major aspects of prevention of injuries and care of the health of the athlete that I feel are fundamental to any sound football program. I would like to emphasize, however, that just *reading* this book about them will not prevent injuries or save lives—it is equally important for all coaches and physicians and trainers to *practice what they know*—to *take action* in all the fundamentals of injury prevention—to insist that the players likewise understand injury prevention and good health practices.

It is hoped that by better understanding of the fundamentals of injury prevention by coaches, physicians, trainers, and players there will be fewer injuries and perhaps even some lives will be saved.

Hundreds of scientific and professional men are devoting many hours of study to ways and means of preventing football injuries and fatalities. This includes not only the medical profession but physiologists, psychologists, trainers, engineers, and others. The American College of Sports Medicine is an organization of professional people whose interest, knowledge, and research in all phases of sports medicine and science are contributing valuable information in this area. The Committee on the Medical Aspects of Sports of the American Medical Association continually makes valuable contributions to our knowledge by their publications, recommendations, and guidelines for team physicians, coaches, and trainers. They sponsor an annual conference for the exchange and exposure of ideas and methods. The American Academy of Orthopaedic Surgeons sponsors excellent symposiums on athletic injuries and publishes many valuable papers on this subject. Other seminars are sponsored by State and County Medical Societies. The National Athletic Trainers Association likewise sponsors meetings and discussion groups for the exchange of ideas, both new and old. The National Federation of State High School Athletic Associations continues to make valuable contributions in the field of health care and injury prevention through their publications and meetings.

Thus it is obvious that action is being taken and progress is being made and the result will certainly be gratifying in terms of fewer serious injuries and healthier and better conditioned athletes.

Chapter 2

THE TEAM PHYSICIAN

SPORTS Medicine is rapidly approaching the category of a true sub-specialty and rightly so, since the knowledge and skills of the physician are needed in safeguarding the health and lives of our young athletes. Some medical schools have instituted courses in the subject; others have set up departments of sports medicine; regional and national seminars are held frequently to help familiarize physicians with problems of prevention and treatment of sports injuries. It is an exciting and rewarding new field for physicians and quite different from the routine of office and hospital practice.

Each school year approximately 25,000 physicians give part- or full-time care to over one million young athletes in junior high, high school, colleges and universities. Most of these physicians serving high schools and smaller colleges give freely of their time, usually without remuneration except in the satisfaction that they are contributing their skills and knowledge in helping to safeguard the health of the young athlete. The information in this chapter is directed mainly to these part-time physicians, especially the newer ones, in an effort to give them an outline of what is expected and how to carry on when they become *Team Physicians.*

How Do You Become a Team Physician? In most of the larger cities, a starting point is to have the President of the County Medical Society appoint a Committee on the Medical Aspects of Sports. This usually is composed of men who are truly interested in the subject and can afford the time to help. The duties of such a committee include furnishing team physicians; holding courses or seminars for physicians, coaches and trainers on the various aspects of sports medicine; and cooperating with the physical education department of the school districts in supervising the health care of the athletes and in discussing various problems in this field that may arise.

In Spokane, Washington, we have always had more than enough volunteer physicians to furnish two team physicians for every high school team. This makes it possible to assure at least one physician in attendance at each game, and frequently one of the pair will attend a practice scrimmage session on his afternoon off. Ideally, a pair of team physicians should consist of an orthopedist or a general surgeon with orthopedic skills, plus a general practitioner, pediatrician, or internist.

In larger towns there are usually a sufficient number of interested and motivated physicians to volunteer for the jobs, particularly if they have a son participating or if they themselves were athletes of greater or lesser fame in their high school and college days.

A major problem exists in providing a physician in attendance for the smaller towns where no physician is practicing. Where these smaller communities are not too far distant from the larger metropolitan areas, some hospitals have furnished interns or residents from their staffs to cover the scheduled games.

There still remain, however, many high school football teams without a team physician and with very little medical supervision or help. It is the hope of all of us who are interested in this aspect of medicine that within the next few years more interested physicians will volunteer their services so that every high school team can have an interested team physician.

The physician does not need a great deal of specialized knowledge to be a team physician for a high school or small college. He must be interested in the players themselves and in the game as it is played. A new team physician should improve his knowledge by reading some of the excellent books on sports medicine, athletic injuries, and care of the athlete, as well as attending some of the excellent seminars on these subjects. (See Appendix for list of publications.)

One enters a rather different world of medicine upon becoming a team physician and at first it is a little strange and slightly bewildering, but interesting and challenging. It seems to me that it took at least two football seasons before I began to feel completely at ease with the coaching staff as well as the players, that I felt confident to give a sensible answer to most questions that were asked, and that I really was contributing something worthwhile.

After a few weeks of association with the coaches and players, the new team physician will be talking about "shin splints," "pinched nerves," "hip-pointers" and other pseudo-scientific terms just as if he had always known about them! He may have to get out the trainer's medical dictionary in the solitude of his den to find out what they mean, but this he will do. He'll learn how to demonstrate the "Louisiana ankle-wrap" as well as if he invented it! The jargon is a little different in the locker room than in the office, but always remember that your presence is always welcome, your knowledge and judgment are always respected, and the coaching staff and players are always proud and happy to have you as a part of the team. You are probably the most important man on the team in safe-guarding a player's health, and without this he ceases to be a player.

What, then, are your main areas of duty as a team physician?

1. First and foremost is the *prevention of injuries*. The most important starting point in prevention of injuries is *proper conditioning* (see Chapter 7). Conditioning, however, must start with a healthy player. Your help in the conditioning program will pertain to advice about diet, sleep, tobacco, alcohol, summer exercising programs, and attaining and maintaining proper weight.

Next to conditioning, the most important aspect in preventing injuries is *good equipment*—your help and advice here can be valuable. Chapter 8 is devoted to equipment.

Most important, your decision as to whether or not to allow a slightly injured player to return to practice or play may be critical in preventing further and more serious injury. Chapters 4 and 5 deal with this aspect.

2. Your second main duty, then is *treatment of injuries*, either by you or by the player's personal or consulting physician. Many fine books have been written on the treatment of athletic injuries (see Appendix) and this subject will not be covered in this book.

3. Lastly, you should make sure the injured player is completely healed and *properly rehabilitated* before allowing him to return to competition.

I would like to emphasize that it is extremely important that the team physician shows enthusiasm and interest in returning the injured athlete to participation as soon as possible and that he *encourages* proper rehabilitation procedures to accomplish this. Occasionally consultation with the player's personal physician will be helpful.

The Pre-season Physical Examination

The best approach to the pre-season physical examination at the high school level is to have it performed by the family physician—who in some cases may also be the team physician. In some schools complete examinations may be done by full-time school physicians. A few important points are worth enumerating here.

1. Examinations should be performed well in advance of the first practice session, preferably in June, but certainly between July 1st and August 1st for football.

2. The old style "line-'em-up-and-run-'em-through" type of physical examination has been long outmoded and is both inadequate and unsatisfactory. A thorough history and complete examination should be performed in the physician's office or other equally suitable quarters.

3. It is acceptable to charge a small fee for the examination, and in many cases some laboratory examinations are indicated. Always do a complete urinalysis.

4. In order to minimize the number of complete physical examinations done on each boy, the following type of schedule has been instituted in many communities:

A. Ideally, a physical examination record form should be completed in duplicate at the time of the first complete examination, usually in the 9th grade. One copy should be given to the parent as a part of the permanent medical record for this player, the other copy kept by the examining physician. This form should have a place for history of serious illnesses, operations, and injuries (especially musculo-skeletal injuries), plus an immunization record. A pamphlet published by the American Medical Association entitled, "A Guide for Medical Evaluation of Candidates for School Sports" is an excellent reference and contains a suggested health examination form.

B. The initial comprehensive examination should be satisfactory through the following year (10th grade), unless the candidate has had a serious intercurrent illness, operation or injury. During the second year a short examination should be sufficient. A card indicating the player's physical fitness should be signed by the examining physician and given to the player to turn in to his coach. This card should list the name, address and telephone number of the physician who is to be called in case of serious injury.

C. At the beginning of the 3rd year (11th grade) another complete examination should be done and this should be made a matter of record as above. This should be sufficient through the senior year except for a short examination again at the start of that year. Thus, two, instead of four complete examinations will ordinarily suffice in the usual healthy young athlete during 9th through 12th grades.

D. The initial examination done at the beginning of the school year should qualify the player for participation in *all* sports for that school year, without need of repeating for each sport he may participate in, unless he has suffered a serious illness or injury since the original examination.

5. The following suggestions will serve as a guide and reminder of some of the aspects of an *examination for sports participation* that ordinarily might be overlooked in a routine type of physical examination:

A. A thorough musculo-skeletal examination should be part of the routine since so many of the injuries in contact sports involve the knee, ankle, shoulder, and spine. Boys with long, lean necks and poor neck musculature are prone to cervical spine injuries. Boys with joint "looseness" or lax ligaments are also more easily injured.

Since the proper procedure for thoroughly and adequately examining the knee is so important, and since some examining physicians who are not orthopedists may not remember the details of a complete knee examination, I am grateful to Dr. Jack Watkins, an eminent orthopedic surgeon with a vast experience in treating knee injuries in athletes, for preparing the following outline.

PROPER PROCEDURE FOR EXAMINATION OF THE KNEES

A short history may give important information:

1. Has the athlete ever suffered a knee injury?
2. Has he ever had a swollen knee—if so, has it recurred?

3. Does the knee ever click when walking or climbing stairs?

4. Has the knee ever locked?

The following examination is a guide to screen out athletes with knee disorders. If there is any question on the following points, the athlete should be referred to an orthopedic surgeon for consultation.

In all knee examinations, *always compare both knees.*

A. With the Athlete Standing.

1. Look for swelling or effusion both anteriorly and posteriorly.

2. Alignment. Does the knee fully extend or hyperextend? Is there excessive bowleg or knock-knee? Does the knee fully flex?

3. With the examiner's hand on the patella, have the athlete do a deep knee bend. (Crepitation usually means significant chondromalacia).

B. With the Athlete Sitting on Table or Bench so that Feet are Not Touching Floor.

1. Check for tenderness along both joint lines to evaluate medial and lateral cartilages and check for tenderness at the site of attachments of both medial and lateral ligaments.

2. Test anterior cruciate ligaments. Place both thumbs on the patella and the fingers of both hands on the back of the upper tibia. *Forcefully* pull the tibia anteriorly while pushing with thumbs against the patella.

3. Test for posterior cruciate ligament. Grasp the upper tibia with both hands and *forcefully* push against the anterior upper tibia. This can also be done with athlete supine and knee flexed 90 degrees.

C. With the Athlete Supine and Relaxed.

1. Medial collateral ligament. Place one hand just above the ankle and raise the entire leg slightly off the table. Place the other hand posteriorly just above the knee and grasp the femoral condyles. With the knee fully extended *force* the knee into valgus (knock-knee). There should be

no significant laxity or opening of the joint on the medial side. Do the same procedure with the knee flexed about 15 degrees. This tests the deep leaf of the medial collateral ligament.

2. Lateral collateral ligament. Using the same technique *force* the knee into varus (bowleg).

3. The "click" of a torn cartilage. Grasp the foot with one hand and place the other hand with thumb over the lateral cartilage and fingers over the medial cartilage. From a position of full extension passively flex the knee to full flexion, at the same time rotating the tibia both internally and externally. A palpable or audible click over the cartilage suggests the possibility of a tear.

4. Atrophy of the thigh muscles is almost always significant if there is ½ inch or more difference in the circumference of the thighs. Measure 6 inches above the upper pole of each patella and place a mark. Measure circumference of each thigh at this point.

The above described examination is not intended for an on-the-field check of a knee, but some of the points can be useful, such as the quick test for instability of the ligaments and range of motion. This is covered in more detail in Chapter 4.

A short but good history is important, with particular emphasis on any recent (12 months) injury or illness which might suggest infectious mononucleosis, hepatitis, renal disease, rheumatic fever, or *bone* or *joint* injury. Are any medications being taken? If so, list them on the examination card.

Every player should have a tetanus toxoid immunization and/or booster (if he has not had a booster within the past 10 years.)

What conditions disqualify a potential athlete for participation in the sport of his choice? The following outline will serve as a guide for the examining physician. You will note that one column lists Relative Contraindications and they are listed this way because (1.) the disability may be mild

CONTACT SPORTS • Football—Wrestling—Baseball—Basketball—Soccer—Rugby—LaCrosse

	Absolute Contraindications	Relative Contraindications
Neurological	1. Concussion with loss of consciousness—out of the game. 2. Two concussions—out for the season. 3. Three concussions—out of contact sports.	1. Epilepsy, if well controlled (no seizure for one year.) 2. A grand mal seizure can follow a head injury without other evidence of epilepsy. This type of seizure should fall into the same category as concussion.
Eye	1. Absence of one eye or amblyopia or one eye 2-/200 (corrected) 2. Retinal detachment (repaired) or (unrepaired) 3. Congenital glaucoma.	1. Active eye infection. 2. Contact lenses—see footnote 1.
Respiratory	1. Any active lung infection, including tuberculosis	1. Bronchial asthma (many participate to tolerance).
Cardiovascular	1. Cardiac enlargement from any cause. 2. Severe mitral stenosis. 3. Aortic stenosis 4. Cyanotic heart disease. 5. Active myocarditis. 6. Symptomatic pulmonary hypertension.	1. Resting BP over 140 systolic and 90 diastolic should be studied before allowing participation.
Endocrine		1. Diabetes is a contraindication only if there is poor control and supervision.
Abdomen	1. Undescended testes over the pubic ramus. 2. Any enlarged major abdominal organ (spleen, liver, kidney)	1. Inguinal hernia.

G.U. System

1. One kidney missing or seriously damaged.
2. Active kidney infection.

1. One testicle missing.

Musculo-skeletal

1. Navicular fracture until healing is complete.
2. Spondylolisthesis and spondylolysis.
3. Hip disease.
   (a) Legg Perthes
   (b) Slipped epiphysis
   (c) Septic hip.
4. Active epiphysitis of the spine.

1. Instability of the knees.
2. Recurrent dislocation of the shoulder.
3. Osgood Schlatter's disease, where there is pain on movement.
4. Tendency to develop myositis ossificans.
5. Amputees—See AMA recommendation footnote 2.

Hematological

1. Blood coagulation defects.

Skin

1. Active bacterial infection
2. Active herpes simplex
3. Severe cystic acne.

Disqualifying Conditions for NON-CONTACT SPORTS—Tennis, Golf, Swimming, Track, Gymnastics

Conditions listed under Contact Sports will apply, with the following exceptions:

	Absolute Contraindications	Relative Contraindications	No Contraindications
Neurological	1. In swimming and certain gymnastics, such as the rings and high bar, epilepsy, if there has been a seizure in the previous year.		1. Susceptibility to cerebral concussion.
Abdomen		1. Enlarged abdominal organ.	
Eye			1. Undescended testes over the ramus.
			1. One eye missing or amblyopic.
Cardiovascular		1. Cardiac enlargement from any cause. 2. Severe mitral stenosis. 3. Aortic stenosis. 4. Active myocarditis. 5. Cyanotic heart disease. 6. Symptomatic pulmonary hypertension. 7. BP above 140/90.	

G.U. System

1. One kidney missing.

1. Testicle missing.

Musculo-skeletal

1. Navicular fracture.

Hematological

1. Blood coagulation defects.

[1]The committee recommends that high school students be urged to use safety lenses in steel frames when participating in contact athletics. Contact lenses have been known to cause serious eye injury from a blow to the eye. Infection under the contact lenses, the frequent loss during play, and the cost of the lenses are important considerations.

[2]*AMA Recommendations for Amputees.*
1. The amputee is otherwise acceptable as a varsity candidate—that is, the only question as to his eligibility for participation is the loss of limb and the prothesis.
2. The integrity of the affected limb is medically affirmed—that is, there is no known underlying bone disease, skin ulceration or other medical contraindications to activity.
3. The decision to play the candidate in competition would not be done for sympathetic or sensational reasons—that is, he would be judged only for his merit compared to his teammate on the basis of training, performance, and sportsmanship.
4. The nature of the specific sport does not impose undue risk for the amputee or the teammates and opponents of the amputee—that is, an inherent risk of the sport does not become a significant risk.

or severe and would have to be individually considered or (2.) participation might be acceptable in one sport but not in another.

DUTIES AND RESPONSIBILITIES

The following outline will serve to give the new team physician a guide to what may be expected from him during the football season. Similar guidelines could be applied to other sports, with modifications.

It should be remembered that in most larger communities, the high school team physician serves in an advisory capacity and refers the treatment of all but minor injuries to the player's family physician, or to specialists as indicated.

Before practice begins, the physician should check over the physical examination records of all the players and if any conditions are noted that suggest further investigation, he should consult with the examining physician.

Physician's Relationship with Coaches and Trainers. 1. He should maintain close liaison with coaches and trainers and feel free to discuss any medical matters with them.

2. He should help and advise the coaching staff in establishing a sound training program. He should assure himself that the coaching staff is thoroughly familiar with the important subjects covered in this book in relation to prevention of injuries, salt and water replacement, heat illness, proper wearing and fitting of good equipment, evaluation of injuries, and all other subjects pertaining to safeguarding the health and lives of the players.

3. He should advise the coaching staff where he or the family physician can be reached in case of a serious injury during practice sessions.

Physician's Relationship with Team Members. 1. He should have full responsibility in recommending that any sick player be temporarily excused from practice sessions until full health is regained.

2. He should follow the general physical status of all

team members, particularly the condition of a previously injured player.

3. Any player who has sustained an injury or illness sufficient to cause him to miss practice for any significant period of time must present a written statement from his personal physician stating he can resume practice. If the team physician disagrees, he should have further consultation with the personal physician regarding the nature and severity of the illness or injury.

4. He should try to be present at several practice sessions per week, especially when a heavy scrimmage is planned.

5. He should be certain that a player with a minor injury does not aggravate it further by continuing to play, either in practice or in games.

Physician's Responsibilities at Game Time. 1. He should be present when the team is warming up before game time and should accompany the team into the dressing rooms between halves.

2. The team physician is to be on the bench with coaches and players.

3. The team physician will go on to the field whenever necessary to evaluate an injury.

4. It is his responsibility and *only his* to make all decisions regarding the removal of an injured player from the game, and whether this player can walk or should be removed on a stretcher. In addition, the physician will decide *whether or not* this injured player may return to the game and when he may return. His authority in this decision must be absolute and unquestioned.

5. He should observe the team carefully when play is in progress to spot players whose behavior is peculiar or abnormal.

6. He should enforce the rule that any injury necessitating an official "time out" means that the injured player must be removed from the game until the physician can assess the extent of his injuries.

7. In case of head or neck injuries, he should be overly

conservative and if there is any evidence of concussion, amnesia, or disorientation, this player should be removed from the game and carefully evaluated. (See Chapter 5— Head and Neck Injuries.)

8. A player with more than a minor injury should be removed to the dressing rooms where the physician can better evaluate the extent of his injury.

9. The team physician should call the player's personal physician when there is any doubt in his mind as to the seriousness or extent of the injury, rendering only necessary and immediate care. (Unless by prior agreement the team physician is also responsible for the treatment of injuries.)

10. At the end of the game he should go into the dressing room and make certain there are no injuries which have not been reported—most frequently there are!

LEGAL ASPECTS OF BEING A TEAM PHYSICIAN

Team physicians, many acting without remuneration, have been sued by parents of minors. A few reminders here may serve to minimize any legal hazards that might befall a part-time team physician.

1. In all cases of players under the age of 21 years, parental permission must be obtained in writing to permit active participation with the team. Equally important the statement must include specific permission for emergency treatment to be given by the team physician in the event of an injury.

2. The team physician has an obligation to act promptly and appropriately in caring for an injured player, first for emergency care and secondly assuring that further definitive care is provided by the physician of choice.

3. If, as team physician, you are unable to be in attendance at a regularly scheduled game, you should provide for medical coverage, making sure that your substitute *will be there*.

4. Legal opinion advises that the physician completing the pre-season physical examination should avoid stating that the boy is "fit for football" or "O.K. for wrestling" or similar statements that might be interpreted legally as guaranteeing a result. It is suggested that the physician state something like "there appears to be no medical reason why this player should not play."

5. Keep records of any treatments you carry out on injured players and retain such records as long as required in your state.

6. If the team physician is also the treating physician, then all the legal implications of the doctor-patient relationship apply.

MINOR ILLNESSES AND SKIN DISORDERS IN ATHLETES

Many athletes, especially in high school, will frequently report for practice when they are suffering from a febrile illness and should properly be home and under treatment. Many of them feel they are "too tough" to forego practice under such circumstances and thus frequently will hide their illness from coach and physician. The team physician should take an active part in educating both the coach and his players about the need for adequate treatment of even the common cold. Lessons to be learned from previous experiences would include:

1. Entire squads have been laid low by a highly contagious *respiratory infection*, particularly when caused by some of the more virulent viruses. The player with the usual upper respiratory infection should be excused from practice until recovery is apparent and until all danger of contagion is over. He should not be allowed in the locker room, or on the playing field—he should be home.

2. Recent reports have indicated that some virus-induced infections may cause *complicating myocarditis*, frequently without symptoms or signs that one might expect. Myocarditis can result in cardiac arrhythmias particularly under

stress of physical exertion and sudden death on the playing field could result. Not only respiratory but gastrointestinal and urological infections have been implicated.

3. *Sore-throats accompanied by fever,* enlarged cervical glands, and general malaise may well be caused by virulent strains of streptococcus or staphylococcus bacteriae. An athlete with such an infection must not be allowed to practice and must be under adequate medical care. The complications are well known and the risk it too great to allow physical activity until recovery is complete.

4. *Skin diseases* are quite frequent in athletes and are often neglected until they become disabling. The team physician should instruct the players and the coach that all skin disorders should be reported at once and examined by a physician to ascertain the cause and advise proper treatment.

A. *Blisters* of the feet are probably the most frequent skin lesions seen in athletes but are readily preventable. When the shoes fit properly and are broken-in properly, blisters rarely occur. In addition, shoes must be kept laced snugly so that no slipping occurs. Avoid putting tincture of benzoin on the feet—it makes them sticky and sticky feet invite blisters. If anything is applied, it should be powder or silicones to allow slippage. Hot-spots, the forerunners of blisters, can be covered with slick tape and the tape coated with grease or powder, thus preventing many blisters from developing.

B. *Contact dermatitis* from tape, elastic bandages, various linaments and ointments used by trainers, lime, chalk, rubber and plastic is quite common. Early attention to such irritants will avoid disabling dermatitis.

C. *Molluscum contagiosum* is seen frequently in wrestlers but can occur in players in other sports. Frequently it is spread by contaminated towels and there should be strict rules about exchange of towels, since other skin conditions including pyoderma can be similarly spread.

D. Trichophytosis or *"athlete's foot"* is common in all athletic squads and steps directed at prevention should include instructions to the players concerning foot hygiene, to include frequent bathing, clean socks once or twice daily, thorough drying between the toes, and the necessary antifungal preparations as prescribed by the team physician. Shower clogs are advised for all members of the squad. Antiseptic foot baths before entering the shower room are useless and may in some cases even be harmful. Fungus infection also can occur in the groin and on the buttocks.

The most important factor in preventing skin infections and their spread to others is cleanliness—both of body and of underclothing and equipment.

Chapter 3

TRAINING ROOM FACILITIES AND MEDICAL EQUIPMENT

$\mathbf{E}$ACH high school and college dressing room area should have a special room designated as a Training Room. It should be isolated from the general dressing room to give some privacy and quiet, should be well lighted, heated, and ventilated. It needs to have a sink with hot and cold running water. Minimal furnishings should include two 7-foot tables, one for taping and one for examinations and dressings; locked cabinet for medical supplies; movable goose-neck type stand lamp; small table and one or two chairs. A small refrigerator or ice machine plus a washer and dryer would make it luxurious.

The Training Room should be stocked with the following:
1. Athletic strapping tape (porous-type)
2. Medical adhesive tape—½", 1", & 2"
3. Tape cutters
4. Band-Aids, ¾" and 1"
5. Sterile gauze squares, all usual sizes
6. Bandage rolls, 2", 3", and 4" of self-adhering type
7. Bandage scissors, large and small

8. Stockinette, 2" and 3"
9. Ace bandages, 2", 3", 4"
10. Cotton balls
11. Roll cotton or cotton batting
12. Sponge rubber
13. Balsa wood splints
14. Splints for arm and leg, both traction type and inflatable plastic type
15. Hand basins, stainless steel
16. Alcohol, rubbing
17. Antibiotic ointment
18. Petrolatum in 1# jars
19. Surgical soap, Liquid Phisohex and bar
20. Antiseptic, Merthiolate
21. Sterile saline in 1 oz. dropper bottle
22. "Heat" or analgesic balm
23. Spirits of ammonia, perles
24. Salt tablets
25. Aspirin tablets
26. Compound tincture of benzoin or "Tough Skin"
27. Foot powder, antiseptic
28. Tongue blades
29. Paper cups
30. Ice packs, chemical type
31. Contact lens solution
32. Sponge-rubber padding, ¼" adhesive type
33. Thermometer, clinical
34. Flash light
35. Ether or tape remover
36. Safety razor and blades
37. One or two books on First Aid for Athletes
38. First Aid Chart for Athletic Injuries, large wall type similar to that on following page. (Available from American Medical Association)
39. If the budget allows:
A. Electric heating pad
B. Infra-red or heat lamp

FIRST AID CHART

FIRST AID, the immediate and temporary care offered to the stricken athlete until the services of a physician can be obtained, minimizes the aggravation of injury and enhances the earliest possible return of the athlete to peak performance. To this end, it is strongly recommended that:

- ALL ATHLETIC PROGRAMS include prearranged procedures for obtaining emergency first aid, transportation, and medical care.
- ALL COACHES AND TRAINERS be competent in first aid techniques and procedures.
- ALL ATHLETES be properly immunized as medically recommended, especially against tetanus and polio.

> Committee on the Medical Aspects of Sports
> AMERICAN MEDICAL ASSOCIATION

To protect the athlete at time of injury,

FOLLOW THESE FIRST STEPS FOR FIRST AID:

STOP play immediately at first indication of possible injury or illness.

LOOK for obvious deformity or other deviation from the athlete's normal structure or motion.

LISTEN to the athlete's description of his complaint and how the injury occurred.

ACT, but move the athlete **only** after serious injury is ruled out.

EMERGENCY PHONE NUMBERS

Physician _____ Phone: _____

Physician _____ Phone: _____

Hospital _____ Ambulance _____

Police _____ Fire _____ Other _____

FOR ATHLETIC INJURIES

BONES AND JOINTS

Fracture—Never move athlete if fracture of back, neck, or skull is suspected. If athlete **can** be moved, carefully splint any possible fracture. Obtain medical care at once.

Dislocation—Support joint. Apply ice bag or cold cloths to reduce swelling, and refer to physician at once.

Bone Bruise—Apply ice bag or cold cloths and protect from further injury. If severe, refer to physician.

Broken Nose—Apply cold cloths and refer to physician.

HEAT ILLNESSES

Heat Stroke—Collapse WITH DRY WARM SKIN indicates sweating mechanism failure and rising body temperature.

THIS IS AN EMERGENCY; DELAY COULD BE FATAL.

Immediately cool athlete by the most expedient means (immersion in cool water is best method). Obtain medical care at once.

Heat Exhaustion Weakness WITH PROFUSE SWEATING indicates state of shock due to depletion of salt and water. Place in shade with head level or lower than body. Give sips of dilute salt water, if conscious. Obtain medical care at once.

Sunburn—If severe, apply sterile gauze dressing; refer to physician.

IMPACT BLOWS

Head—If any period of dizziness, headache, incoordination, or unconsciousness occurs, disallow any further activity and obtain medical care at once. Keep athlete lying down; if unconscious, give nothing by mouth.

Teeth—Save teeth if completely removed from socket. If loosened, do not disturb; cover with sterile gauze and refer to dentist at once.

Celiac Plexus—Rest athlete on back and moisten face with cool water. Loosen clothing around waist and chest. Do nothing else except obtain medical care if needed.

Testicle—Rest athlete on back and apply ice bag or cold cloths. Obtain medical care if pain persists.

Eye—If vision is impaired, refer to physician at once. With soft tissue injury, apply ice bag or cold cloths to reduce swelling.

MUSCLES AND LIGAMENTS

Bruise—Apply ice bag or cold cloths, and rest injured muscle. Protect from further aggravation. If severe, refer to physician.

Cramp—Have opposite muscles contracted forcefully, using firm hand pressure on cramped muscle. If during hot day, give sips of dilute salt water. If recurring, refer to physician.

Strain and Sprain—Elevate injured part and apply ice bag or cold cloths. Apply pressure bandage to reduce swelling. Avoid weight bearing and obtain medical care.

OPEN WOUNDS

Heavy Bleeding—Apply sterile pressure bandage using hand pressure if necessary. Refer to physician at once.

Cut and Abrasion—Hold briefly under cold water. Then cleanse with mild soap and water. Apply sterile pad firmly until bleeding stops, then protect with more loosely applied sterile bandage. If extensive, refer to physician.

Puncture Wound—Handle same as cuts, and refer to physician.

Nose bleed—Keep athlete sitting or standing; cover nose with cold cloths. If bleeding is heavy, pinch nose and place **small** cotton pack in nostrils. If bleeding continues, refer to physician.

OTHER CONCERNS

Blisters—Keep clean with mild soap and water and protect from aggravation. If already broken, trim ragged edges with sterilized equipment. If extensive or infected, refer to physician.

Foreign Body in Eye—Do not rub. Gently touch particle with point of clean, moist cloth and wash with cold water. If unsuccessful or if pain persists, refer to physician.

Lime Burns—Wash thoroughly with water. Apply sterile gauze dressing and refer to physician.

Prepared by the AMA Committee on the Medical Aspects of Sports in cooperation with the National Athletic Trainers Association and the National Federation of State High School Athletic Associations. (Reprinted with Permission)

THE EMERGENCY MEDICAL BAG

Each athletic squad should have at least one good emergency bag which is well constructed and is weather proof. It should be completely stocked and checked thoroughly before each practice session and game. It should be on the field at each practice session and each game.

The emergency bag should be stocked with at least the following items; the team physician may add other items he deems necessary.

1. Adhesive tape
2. Strapping tape
3. Sterile gauze squares
4. Bandage rolls, self-adhering type
5. Ace bandages
6. Cotton balls
7. Rubbing alcohol
8. Bandage scissors
9. Razor and blades
10. Tongue blades
11. Plastic airway
12. Tongue forceps
13. Stethoscope and sphygmomanometer
14. Tincture of benzoin
15. Petroleum jelly
16. Normal saline in dropper bottle
17. Aspirin
18. Ice packs, chemical type
19. Flash light
20. Splints, plastic inflatable type
21. Otoscope and ophthalmoscope.

PLAYING FIELD EQUIPMENT

The following important items should be present on the playing field, particularly during a game to insure adequate management of the injured player:

1. The emergency medical bag
2. A portable litter—Army type or comparable

3. A plywood-board litter—¾" or thicker plywood with four handles bolted to the board. This is *always* used in moving an injured player who is suspected of having sustained a spinal cord injury. The canvas or plastic type stretcher sags too much to afford rigidity necessary in moving the player with the above type of injury.

4. Blankets for the litter with plastic cover.

5. Four sandbags, approximately 12" x 6" in size (for immobilizing neck or extremity injuries.)

6. Ambulance, or station wagon, large enough to transport injured player on stretcher.

The following items should be available for comfort, replacement, and repair:

1. Waterproof parkas and/or blankets for each member of the squad, including the coaching staff and team physician.

2. Benches for the players and be sure they use them! Squad members standing on the sidelines are hazardous to the players, obstruct vision of spectators, and suggest disorganization.

3. Spare laces for shoes and shoulder pads; spare chin straps.

4. Spare jerseys.

5. One extra set of contact lens for every player that uses them. (Have you ever tried to find a lost contact in the heat of battle? They are rarely found!)

6. Water—fresh and cold—in suitable containers with either spigot outlets or pressure-type spray outlets.

7. Paper cups for *individual—not group*—use.

8. Towels—clean and dry cloth towels, plus paper towels.

STUDENT MANAGERS AND TRAINERS

Managers and/or trainers of high school and small college teams are usually boys who enjoy athletics but may not have the size or ability to make the squad. They are dedicated errand boys for the coaching staff and valets for the athletes. In addition, however, they frequently are expected to assume a responsible position in caring for minor aches and pains, skin abrasions and lacerations, and other minor injuries. Many times they have received no formal training for this responsibility. To this end, every effort should be made to train these boys as adequately as possible.

1. All trainers and managers should be qualified Red Cross First Aid trainees. Short of this, they should be familiar with the principles and practice of first aid.

2. Some school districts have set up training courses for student managers administered by graduate trainers, team physicians, and other qualified personnel. All schools should provide student trainers with such courses.

3. The team physician can teach the student trainer many fundamentals, especially in the field of what *not* to do.

4. Many splendid books are available and should be part of the training room equipment (see Appendix).

5. It is extremely important that the team physician sit down with the coaches and all trainers before the season begins to establish exactly which injuries must be seen by a doctor immediately and which injuries can safely wait until the boy can see his doctor after practice. Many minor injuries do not require the attention of a physician and can be adequately handled by the coach or trainer. The important point is to advise exactly what injuries cannot be handled by the trainer and must be evaluated by the physician.

Chapter 4

EXAMINATION OF THE INJURED
ATHLETE ON THE FOOTBALL FIELD

THE immediate examination of the injured athlete on the football field to determine the degree and extent of injury is of utmost importance. Many high school team physicians are not orthopedists and consequently do not usually deal with traumatic musculo-skeletal injuries as often as their orthopedic colleagues. For this reason a review of the most important points in such an examination will contribute to their knowledge and skill.

At the Fifth National Conference on the Medical Aspects of Sports held in Portland, Oregon, in 1963, Dr. Martin E. Blazina, orthopedic surgeon and team physician for the University of California at Los Angeles, presented a most outstanding, concise, and informative paper on the proper technique for examining the injured football player on the field. The paper subsequently was published in the Proceedings of the Fifth National Conference on the Medical Aspects of Sports, published by the American Medical Association.

I am very grateful to Dr. Blazina and the AMA for their permission to reprint this excellent article.

DEVELOPING A PROPER TECHNIQUE FOR EXAMINING THE INJURED ATHLETE ON THE FOOTBALL FIELD
AN OUTLINE FOR THE TEAM PHYSICIAN

The development of a proper technique for examining the injured athlete on the football field depends upon:

• An understanding of the responsibilities of the physician on the playing field;

• Adequate preparation for carrying out these responsibilities;

• Utilization of sound general principles as guideposts in the examination; and

• Involvement of simple logical approaches in the diagnosis of certain specific types of injuries.

I. Responsibilities of the team physician on the playing field.

A. The team physician should disallow further participation when an injury has been sustained *that could be detrimental to the athlete's future well-being* (even though he is apparently performing satisfactorily). For example, the player who has performed excellently in the first half but who has noticed hematuria during the half-time recess should not return to the game.

B. The team physician should disallow further participation when an injury has been sustained *that interferes significantly with the effectiveness of the player's performance* (even though the injury is not potentially serious in itself). Inability to perform satisfactorily could lead to aggravation of the original injury or could be responsible for a secondary, more serious injury. Also, if the athlete is unable to maintain his usual standard of performance, it would be of more benefit to the team for him to be replaced. For example, any injury of the lower extremity which causes the player to limp noticeably should be cause for withdrawal from the game.

C. The team physician should allow and encourage further participation when an injury has been sustained *that is not potentially serious and does not interfere significantly with the effectiveness of the athlete's performance.* This important responsibility sometimes is overlooked. This approach teaches the athlete to continue competition despite a minor physical setback and also does not deprive the team of his potential contributions. For example, a contusion of the shin may be painful, but if, in the opinion of the team physician, a more serious type of injury is unlikely, and if the athlete is able to run and jump normally, he should be allowed to continue.

II. Adequate preparation for carrying out the team physician's responsibilities on the football field.

A. *Being prepared to perform a complete and competent examination as soon as possible after the injury.* An incomplete and incompetent examination leads to diagnostic errors. Proper treatment depends upon proper diagnosis. The initial examination immediately after the mishap may reveal findings which become obscured after a relatively short time.

B. *Making prior arrangements for emergency first aid on the playing field.* All too often, basic equipment such as stretchers and splints are not available at the time of injury.

C. *Making prior arrangements for further diagnostic and therapeutic measures at a nearby medical facility.* Expeditious transfer enhances the standard of care and helps allay apprehension for all concerned.

D. *Making prior arrangements to obtain expert consultation when required.* The field of athletic medicine is too vast to be encompassed by a single physician and he should have in mind whom to call for special situations.

E. *Having a prior knowledge of the participants if possible.* This makes for accurate appraisal of injuries and avoids errors in diagnosis.

F. *Making one's presence known to the coaches and offi-*

cials. A game should not start until it has been noted that a team physician is present on the field.

G. *Being available in the dressing room after the game.* Approximately 50 per cent of the injuries incurred during a game are first noted after play has discontinued. This is also the time to begin treatment, not the following Monday.

III. Sound general principles to be used as guideposts in the examination of the injured athlete.

A. *Listen (to a description of)*

1. The mechanism of injury. How did the injury happen? Were you hit? With what?

2. The complaints. What is the matter? How does the injury bother you?

3. The area of localization of pain. Where do you hurt? Is that where you were hit?

B. *Look (and feel) for*

1. Deformity: Always a sign of a significant injury.

2. Swelling: Aids in localizing the problem and should be controlled to facilitate recovery.

3. Defects ⎫
           ⎬ Indicate a definite injury.
4. Crepitus ⎭

5. Areas of tenderness: Also aid in localization and diagnosis. Determine if intra-articular or extra-articular.

6. Instability: Always check opposite side and ask about past injuries.

7. Loss of motion: An important finding before spasm occurs.

8. Loss of function: Always indicates a signficant injury, if a true finding.

C. *Stop (and)*

1. Rule out the most serious injury first, then go on to a more specific diagnosis.

2. Use a stretcher if needed. It takes only a few minutes and avoids added discomfort.

3. Reconsider before unnecessarily moving a player with a possible neck injury.

4. Complete examination before allowing a player to return to the game, no matter how long it takes.

5. Do not apply ice packs or tight wraps if the player may possibly return to the game.

6. Reconsider before telling an injured player that he has a potentially serious injury.

IV. Simple logical approaches in the diagnosis and treatment of certain specific types of injuries.

A. HEAD INJURIES

Findings	Return	No Return
1. Unconscious ("10 second count")		x
2. Saw stars or colors		x
3. One side of body feels numb		x
4. Momentarily dazed	?	?
5. Dizzy		x
6. Severe headache		x
7. Abnormal pupils		x
8. Amnesia		x
9. Disoriented		x
10. Lethargic		x
11. Hyperirritable		x

Considerations

• Be on the alert for other injuries, especially neck injuries.

• If a player is only momentarily dazed and has absolutely no other findings, the team physician may consider returning him to the game.

• However, if there are any other findings, he absolutely should not be returned to the game.

B. NECK INJURIES

Findings	Return	No Return
1. Obvious deformity of neck		x
2. Tenderness a) over cervical spinous processes		x
b) over upper thoracic spinous processes	?	?
c) over trapezius	?	?
d) over sternocleidomastoid	?	?
3. Restricted motion of neck		x
4. Weakness of extremities		x
5. Numbness of extremities		x
6. Pain radiating down the arm	?	?

Considerations
- Always check for a concomitant head injury.
- If the player has no restriction of motion, no deformity, no neurological symptoms or superficial tenderness over the cervical musculature or the upper thoracic spinous processes, then only should one consider returning him to the game.
- Conservatism should be the rule.
- X-ray pictures should be taken in all cases where there is the slightest doubt about the seriousness of the injury.

C. ABDOMINAL INJURIES

Findings	Return	No Return
1. Wind knocked out	x	
2. Nauseated		x
3. Dizzy—faint—shocky		x
4. Tenderness Superficial	x	
Deep		x

Considerations
- Be very suspicious of a possible ruptured spleen if there has been a recent history of infectious mononucleosis.
- If a player has had his wind knocked out and has only superficial tenderness (that is, involving the abdominal musculature), he may return to the game.
- However, if he has a deep tenderness (that is, intraperitoneal or retroperitoneal) or is nauseated or shocky, he definitely should not return to the game.

D. SHOULDER INJURIES

Findings		Return	No Return
1. Obvious deformity	a) Sternoclavicular joint		x
	b) Shaft of clavicle		x
	c) Acromioclavicular joint		x
	d) Glenohumeral joint		x
2. Tenderness	a) Sternoclavicular joint	?	
	b) Shaft of clavicle	?	
	c) Acromioclavicular joint	?	
	d) Trapezius	?	
	e) Deltoid	?	
	f) Rotator cuff	?	
3. Crepitus	a) Sternoclavicular joint		x
	b) Shaft of clavicle		x
	c) Acromioclavicular joint		x
	d) Glenohumeral joint		x
4. "Spring"	a) Sternoclavicular joint		x
	b) Acromioclavicular joint		x
5. Shoulder "slipped out."			x

Considerations

● Always remove the jersey and shoulder pads for a complete examination.

● If there is a combination of tenderness plus another finding (that is, deformity, crepitus, or instability), then the player should not return to the game.

● "Shoulder slipping out" indicates a probable subluxation of the shoulder and should be treated exactly like a frank dislocation.

E. KNEE INJURIES

	Findings	Return	No Return
1. Obvious deformity	a) Tibiofemoral dislocation		x
	b) Dislocated patella		x
	c) Dislocated head of fibula		x
2. Defect	a) Quadriceps tendon		x
	b) Patella		x
	c) Patellar tendon		x
	d) Tibial tubercle		x
	e) At lateral joint line		x
	f) At hamstring insertions		x
	g) Head of fibula		x
	h) Medial femoral condyle		x
	i) Medial joint line		x
	j) At or near pes anserinus		x
3. Crepitus	a) Patella		x
	b) Head of fibula		x
	c) At joint line		x
	d) Medial femoral condyle		x
4. Tenderness	a) Quadriceps tendon	?	
	b) Patella	?	
	c) Patellar tendon	?	
	d) Tibial tubercle	?	
	e) Lateral joint line	?	
	f) Hamstring insertions	?	
	g) Lateral femoral condyle	?	
	h) Head of fibula	?	
	i) Medial femoral condyle	?	
	j) Medial joint line	?	
	k) Over or near pes anserinus	?	
	l) Popliteal region	?	

E. KNEE INJURIES (continued)

	Findings	Return	No Return
5. Range of motion	a) Loss of active extension		x
	b) Loss of active flexion		x
	c) Loss of passive extension		x
	d) Loss of passive flexion		x
6. Stability	a) Laxity of medial collateral ligament		x
	b) Laxity of lateral collateral ligament		x
	c) Positive anterior drawer sign		x
	d) Positive posterior drawer sign		x
7. "Knee cap felt as if it slipped out."			x
8. "Knee went out."			x

Considerations
- Use the other knee for comparison and ask about other injuries.
- Tenderness plus another finding should lead to disallowing further participation.
- Definite localization of tenderness and its proper notation may lead to more accurate diagnosis and aids surgery if it is ever contemplated.

F. ANKLE INJURIES

Findings		Return	No Return
1. Obvious dislocation or deformity			x
2. Defect	a) Beneath tip of medial malleolus		x
	b) Beneath tip of lateral malleolus		x
3. Crepitus	a) Medial malleolus		x
	b) Lateral malleolus		x
	c) Anywhere along length of fibula		x
4. Tenderness	a) Medial aspect of ankle	?	
	b) Anterior aspect of ankle	?	
	c) Lateral aspect of ankle	?	
	d) Posterior aspect of ankle	?	
	e) Anywhere along length of fibula	?	
	f) Over peroneal tendons	?	
5. Swelling	a) Over region of calcaneo-fibular ligament		x
	b) Over region of anterior talofibular ligament		x
	c) Over region of deltoid ligament		x
6. Range of motion	a) Increased inversion		x
	b) Increased eversion		x
	c) Increased anteroposterior motion		x
7. "Spring" to ankle mortise			x

Considerations

• Tenderness plus another finding should lead to withdrawal from the game.

• Always check the fibula along its entire length up to the fibula head for every ankle injury.

• Always check the foot for every ankle injury.

• Swelling may be quite rapid.

• Check tendon function and tendon position (especially the peroneal tendons and heel cord).

Chapter 5

HEAD AND NECK INJURIES—Their Prevention, Evaluation, and Immediate Care

SINCE head and neck injuries are the leading causes of death from football injuries, and since many of these tragic deaths could be prevented if all coaches, trainers, and physicians were familiar with the factors involved, this chapter is devoted in some detail to discussing practices which may help prevent some of these fatal injuries. It is extremely important that the coach and team physician have a well-planned and predetermined course of action in order to evaluate and manage the player who sustains an injury to the head, neck, or spine. There is no intention here of telling the physician exactly what he should or should not do, but the following suggestions should serve as valuable guidelines to both coach and team physician.

Since 1960, most of the direct fatalities in football have been caused by head and neck injuries. In 1968 *all* of the direct fatalities were the result of head and neck injuries and in 1969, 84% of the fatalities were due to such injuries.

Thus the prevention of head and neck injuries assumes major importance in saving lives.

In reviewing the cumulative statistics on direct fatalities since 1931, the following conclusions should be significant to all high school coaches:

1. About 55% of the fatalities occurred among players between 16 and 18 years of age—the high school player.

2. Almost 50% occurred during regularly scheduled games.

3. Almost 33% of the fatal injuries occurred to the player when he was tackling his opponent.

4. About 16% occurred to the player when carrying the ball.

5. About 10% occurred to the player who was blocking.

6. Defensive players have slightly more fatal injuries than offensive players.

By comparison, an astounding increase in fatal injuries in football occurred in 1968—36 direct fatalities, more than double the per-year average for 1931 to 1964! Admittedly, there were more players participating in 1968, but the figure also represents a higher percentage. In high school football the incidence of fatal injuries per 100,000 players was 1.63 per year for 1931 to 1964, but 2.6 in 1968. In college players it was 2.52 per 100,000 players for 1931 to 1964, but was 6.6 in 1968. *In 1968 all of the direct fatalities were the result of injuries to the head, neck, and spinal cord!*

One other significant observation from these statistics—almost one-third of the fatal injuries occurred to the player when he was tackling the opponent, less than half of this number during ball carrying, and about 10% when blocking.

By comparison, however, football is actually not a high-risk activity, as regards fatal injuries. Nine times as many young men die in automobile accidents per man-hour of exposure as die on the football field.

PREVENTION OF HEAD AND NECK INJURIES

The coach, trainer, and physician can together carry out certain procedures which will serve to prevent many serious head and neck injuries. There is no way to prevent *all* of them, but certainly every effort must be taken to reduce the incidence and severity of these potentially fatal injuries.

Many important studies have been made in both high schools and colleges of the causes and mechanisms of head and neck injuries. Important conclusions can be made from these studies, some of which can help to prevent such injuries.

1. In an important study done on high school players, Dr. Richard H. Alley, Jr.,* of Pasadena, California, reported that *only 4.7%* of all the players receiving head injuries were wearing properly fitted helmets. Another 19.6% had helmets fitted inadequately. The remainder wore *very poorly* fitted helmets (75.7%)!

Conclusion—A good helmet, well-fitted, properly worn, and frequently inspected for suspension, cracks, or other damage is most important. The helmet that is not fitted snugly around the head with proper adjustment of suspension straps will offer little or no help in dispersion and absorption of the blow to the head.

2. Since most head injuries result from impact of the player's head against the opponent's knee (about 35%); the opponent's helmet (about 25%); or the turf (about 15%); certain recommendations can be made:

A. In probably one-third of all head and neck injuries a basic fundamental of football play is usually violated. These would include having the head down and neck flexed at the time of contact, and tackling at knee level or below.

B. In this study it was found that about 60% of head injuries and 44% of neck injuries occurred in players who were coached to "spear." Some were instructed to spear in tackling as well as in blocking. When the spearing was taught so as to hit the opponent below the belt with the helmet, the head frequently came in contact with the opponent's knee.

*Journal of the American Medical Association, May 4, 1964, p. 118.

Conclusion—Spearing must not be taught and, further, must be outlawed.

In addition, the player must be properly coached to strike his opponent with his forehead and face bar with his *head up*—and be continuously warned against ducking his head on contact and thus butting his opponent or hitting him with the top of his helmet. This is when the serious injuries can occur, because of the chance of acute flexion of the head and neck.

C. Since over one-third of head injuries and many neck injuries result when the player's head strikes the opponent's knee or thigh, it is obvious that the running knee is a dangerous weapon.

Conclusion—steps should be taken to improve the padding about the knee in order to reduce the impact force, thus both helping to prevent injury to the head and neck, as well as minimizing contusions to the knee and thigh.

D. Further efforts are being made to design a helmet which has some external padding of a resilient material which would further help in absorbing and distributing the force of the impact, as well as to make the helmet a less dangerous weapon when striking the opponent.

3. This same study on head and neck injuries in high school athletes reported that in 72% of the players receiving *head* injuries, *less than 7 days* had been spent in preseason conditioning before beginning scrimmage; that in 81% of players receiving *neck* injuries, less than 7 days had been spent in team conditioning, and even worse, in 10% practice was begun before *any* group conditioning had been carried out.

In this same group it was reported that for over 50% of the players sustaining neck injuries, less than 3 minutes daily was spent in neck-strengthening exercises.

Conclusion—Preseason conditioning can never be overlooked as the number one factor in preventing such injuries, with adequate time spent on exercises to strengthen necks.

4. It has been noted that about 5% of all cerebral concussions occur on the kick-off play—a relatively high incidence for such a brief moment of activity.

Conclusion—Some steps might be taken to lessen the dangers in this situation.

5. In college football studies of head injuries, it was shown that about 45% of all players sustaining head injuries had histories of prior episodes of head injuries in the same or preceding years. Figures for high school players would probably be considerably less, since in many cases boys who sustain head injuries are well advised to switch to non-contact sports.

Conclusion—If you have players who seem to be prone to head injuries, it would be wise to make certain they are fitted with the best available protective helmet and that all precautions are taken to be sure that this helmet is fitted properly to afford the most protection. If a high school player sustains three concussions and/or contusions, he should give up contact sports for his lifetime.

EVALUATING SEVERITY OF
HEAD INJURIES ON THE FIELD

The player sustaining an injury sufficient to cause unconsciousness or semi-consciousness for even a brief period must be carefully evaluated *on the field* before undertaking to remove him to the sidelines. Unconsciousness will most often be related to a head injury, but in rare instances trauma to the cervical spine can cause unconsciousness.

1. Note the length of time of unconsciousness—the longer duration *usually* indicates more severe injury. However, relatively minor head blows with only dazing have been followed by intracranial bleeding, so follow-up observation is very important.

2. Check the dazed player on the spot for his memory recall of events just preceding the head blow—what day is it, what position was he playing, what was the play, whom did he hit, what period is it, what is the score? Prolonged

periods of memory loss are usually associated with more severe injuries.

3. Is he dizzy or unsteady? Does he have ringing in his ears or noises in his head? Again, the extent and severity of such symptoms are related to the degree of injury, usually.

4. Look at his pupils—are they equal in size? Any obvious inequality of pupil size is usually a serious sign and the player should be seen by a physician immediately.

5. If, after careful evaluation, it is obvious that the player has sustained a head injury, then, depending upon the duration and degree of unconsciousness, the patient can be removed from the field as follows:

A. If the patient has had only a momentary lapse of consciousness and is only slightly dazed, after regaining consciousness he can be helped off the field by one or two aides without use of a stretcher.

B. If after 2 to 3 minutes a player has not regained sufficent consciousness and strength to stand upright and walk, he should *always* be moved from the playing field via stretcher. *Never* make the mistake of dragging a *semi-conscious* player off the field on his feet.

C. If complete unconsciousness is prolonged—over 2 to 3 minutes—then the patient should be removed via stretcher to the sidelines where the team physician, or in his absence the coach, can further and carefully evaluate the extent of the head injury.

D. In moving the unconscious player with possible severe *head* injury (*not neck injury*), certain precautions should be taken:

1. Place him on the stretcher *on his side* in order to maintain a clear airway and also to allow secretions and vomitus to drain from his mouth.

2. A plastic airway may have to be inserted to maintain unobstructed airway if his breathing seems labored.

3. If no physician is immediately available, get him in an ambulance or station wagon and to the hospital at once.

The player who seemingly has recovered consciousness rapidly and is sitting on the bench should be continuously observed by a well-trained attendant for further recovery or further development of symptoms. Any notation of increasing signs or symptoms as noted above should be evaluated immediately by the physician. In addition to those above, the player may develop severe headache, nausea and vomiting. These *may* indicate intracranial bleeding.

EVALUATING THE SEVERITY OF NECK OR BACK INJURIES ON THE FIELD

The most important point in evaluating such an injury is to determine whether there has been a fracture and/or dislocation of a vertebra, and, *most important*, an accompanying *spinal cord injury*. A brief neurological evaluation must be done before any attempt is made to move the player and this should be done by the physician. However, in his absence, the coach and trainer can get some idea of the severity and extent of the injury by observing the following points.

1. Usually the player with a spinal cord injury will not be unconscious, but occasionally severe cervical (neck) cord injuries will cause unconsciousness.

2. Ask about pain—what part of the neck or lower spine is affected? Is there pain down the arms? Is there tenderness over the injured area?

3. Can he move all his extremities—feet, legs, hands, and arms? If so, the chances of a severe spinal cord injury are slight. Is there muscle weakness in any extremity?

4. Does he have numbness or tingling in any part of his body. If not, again the chances of a severe spinal cord injury are lessened.

5. Is he able to rotate his head from side to side or is it locked to one side? Locking usually indicates serious injury.

6. Fractures of the spine can occur without obvious spinal cord injury so that the absence of the signs enumerated

above does *not* rule out fracture. If there is the slightest doubt, conclude that he has fractured his spine until proven otherwise.

7. If, after careful evaluation of the severity of the injury as noted above, there is the slightest evidence that there *could* be an injury to the vertebrae and/or spinal cord, the utmost precautions must be taken in moving the injured player to prevent additional damage.

A. Neck Injury

1. The patient should be turned carefully on his back, using four or five persons to do this, with one person maintaining the neck in neutral position (preventing side-to-side or rotary motion) with traction. If proper traction is maintained, it is highly unlikely that further injury would be produced.

2. Carefully then place the patient on his back on the inflexible (plywood or equivalent) stretcher, maintaining neck traction consistently.

3. Sand bags can then be applied to each side of the head and neck with manual traction being maintained.

4. This meticulous handling must be maintained into the hospital and into the x-ray room until the physician responsible for the complete care of the patient takes over.

B. Dorsal or Lumbar Spine Injury.

Suspected fracture or fracture-dislocations of the dorsal or lumbar spine also require that the patient be moved cautiously to the firm stretcher in either the supine or prone position. Do not allow the player to sit up, turn or flex.

FOLLOW-UP CARE IN CASE OF HEAD INJURIES

1. Head injury sufficient to cause only momentary unconsciousness or disorientation comprises by far the largest group and is a fairly frequent occurrence. However, one must remember that occasionally an apparently relatively minor trauma to the head has resulted in later internal cranial bleeding. The patient who recovers complete neuro-

logical function both mentally and physically following this momentary period of unconsciousness should be carefully observed for the next 24 hours, preferably in an infirmary or hospital. However, sometimes this is not possible or accepted by the patient or parents, and in this case the physician should instruct the parents to make periodic checks of the boy's condition for the next 24 hours.

A. Awaken him every hour to be sure he can be aroused and is not unconscious.

B. Make sure he can move all extremities.

C. Question him about headache, visual disturbance, or nausea.

D. Check for inequality of size of pupils.

E. If any unusual signs or symptoms occur (even after 24 hours), immediate medical attention is needed for proper evaluation and diagnosis.

If no unusual symptoms or signs have occurred after 24 hours, the player should under no circumstances return to contact sports for a period of at least 1 week.

2. Head injury causing unconsciousness that is more than momentary, and prolonged (more than a few minutes) loss of memory for recent events, indicates the player has likely sustained some degree of contusion to the brain. He may also complain of persistent headache, nausea, vomiting, show unsteadiness or other neurological signs. All such patients should be hospitalized and a complete neurological work-up performed by the personal physician.

If, after complete neurological study, his symptoms abate and recovery is uncomplicated, this athlete should refrain from any type of sports activity for *at least 2 weeks.*

3. The most serious head injuries are usually those associated with prolonged unconsciousness and skull fractures and/or intracranial bleeding. These obviously require immediate hospitalization and skilled neurological care.

An athlete who has recovered from a skull fracture and/ or intracranial bleeding should forego any further participation in contact sports *during his lifetime.*

4. One further observation is in order. Certain high school athletes seem to be unable to weather head blows very well without suffering varying periods of unconsciousness and prolonged headaches following such trauma, although these prove to be only concussion or mild contusion. It is generally recommended that any boy who has experienced three or more such episodes during his career in contact sports should give up contact sports in favor of non-contact sports.

5. Athletes who have sustained any significant injury to the cervical spine should never again participate in contact sports, or diving.

The electroencephalogram is most valuable in determining extent of damage and aiding the physician's decision as to further participation of any athlete with a head injury.

Chapter 6

THE COACH—His Responsibilities in Preventing Injuries

THE coach is the No. 1 man in protecting the health and safety of the athlete. His ability in teaching the athlete how to perform skillfully will be a significant factor in lowering the incidence and decreasing the severity of injuries. This chapter will point out some of the ways in which the coach can best fulfill his duties in safeguarding the health of his players and preventing injuries.

1. The coach must make certain that every player has *completed his physical examination* and has a signed card from the examining physician *before the first practice session* begins. This should be a hard-and-fast rule, with no exceptions.

2. The coach should individually and carefully *evaluate each new boy* who is turning out for the team by means of a *short personal interview.*

In addition, ideally, the head coach should meet with the parents of each new boy and discuss the football program. This should enable him to evaluate the boy from the physical and psychological standpoint, noting his apparent fitness, type of build, relative maturity, general motivation, and perhaps discussing any personal problems the boy may have as regards athletic competition.

Equally important, the coach should be familiar with the scholastic background of each new player, which would include information concerning his previous school grades, conduct, attitude, work habits, and attendance record. Such an interview not only helps the coach but may give the boy a feeling of security, of belonging, and of a greater desire to do well. Such an interview also proves that the coach is sincerely concerned about the physical and emotional health of his players.

3. It is extremely important that the coach takes extra time and effort to *match the younger players* turning out for the Freshman and/or B Squads. Not only should they be matched by height and weight, but consideration must be given to muscular development, coordination, agility, and skill. It is during this age of rapid growth that a great danger of injury exists. In addition this is frequently an age of emotional sensitivity during which time thoughtless criticism by coaches or parents or inadequate recognition of their potential abilities and efforts can result in discouragement and indifference.

4. The high school coach can help in preventing injuries if he carefully *evaluates his squad from the standpoint of physical strength, agility, and skill* when he chooses certain boys for their positions on the team, be it defense or offense. He should know that the defensive ends, the cornerback spot, the tight end, the pulling guards, and the halfbacks are the most vulnerable to injury and the boys playing these spots have to be sturdy and strong.

5. *Insurance.* The coach must be certain that an adequate insurance program is in force before the first practice session starts and that it includes coverage for general bodily injury as well as *dental* injuries.

Since many times there is some delay in *individual* insurance coverage due to various factors, it has proven wise to ask the school to take out a blanket insurance policy covering *all* players for the first 2 or 3 weeks of practice. This provides coverage for some players who might drop out after a few days of practice or some who might delay personal payment of their insurance when this is required.

6. The coaches must personally be sure that the squad has *good protective equipment* and that each player has individual instruction and help in properly fitting and wearing this protective equipment. (See Chapter 8 on Equipment.)

7. The coach and his staff must *inspect the practice and playing fields* before play begins to make certain that they are in safe condition, which includes freedom from holes, debris such as rocks, glass, tin cans, old boards; that fixed objects on the field are not too close to the sidelines; and that practice equipment is not left in a hazardous spot. In many instances he may have to supervise the ground-keeping too, seeing that the turf is kept in as good a condition as possible by frequent watering, mowing, and cleaning. In addition, the coach should insist that the locker room be kept in a clean condition at all times. A good student manager can be assigned the duty and responsibility of field inspection and maintenance to be done each afternoon before practice begins. Another student manager should be responsible for locker room maintenance.

8. *Proper conditioning* of the athlete is the most important factor in the prevention of injuries. The coaching staff that spends too little time on conditioning will regret this haste as the season progresses. Since proper conditioning is such a vital matter in prevention of athletic injuries, this subject is discussed in detail in the following chapter.

9. A good coach must learn to *recognize and evaluate injuries* in the absence of the team physician, which at the high school and small college level may be frequent, especially during practice. He must be *over-conservative* in all

instances and use the utmost precautions in evaluating head and neck injuries, extremity injuries, and abdominal injuries. He must learn the proper technique in moving injured players with potentially serious injuries. (See Chapter 5 on Head and Neck Injuries.) He must not hesitate to call the team physician or the player's family physician and the player's parents in an instance of a potentially dangerous injury. He must be sure that there is available at all times proper equipment for moving the injured player and that an ambulance can be called for emergency services.

10. A good coach will know the rules outlined in Chapter 7 about *practicing in the heat*, realizing that most cases of heat stroke and/or heat exhaustion occur during the first 2 weeks of practice, especially in August heat.

11. A coach must never take the *responsibility for the technical medical care of any injury*—this is the duty of the team physician, or of the player's family physician.

12. The coach must accept the team *physician's decisions* in all matters pertaining to players' injuries as final and absolute. He must abide by the medical decision as to when and if the player may return to practice; if and when he may return to a game in which he has been injured; and in some instances if the boy should cease further participation. There must be mutual respect between coach and team physician at all times. The relative seriousness of injuries should be discussed privately between coach and physician.

13. The coach who can afford a *professional trainer* is indeed fortunate, since this immediately relieves him of many responsibilities regarding injuries, treatment, proper rehabilitation. However, at the high school level most trainers are student trainers who pick up their knowledge from the senior student trainers and try to learn as much as possible from reading and observation. In such cases, it is most important that at the start of the season the coach, team physician, and student trainers have several sessions during which the physician must advise the trainers concerning first aid treatments, treatment of minor injuries, and most

important to instruct the student trainers on *what not to do.* Telephone consultations from the coach to the team physician concerning injuries during practice sessions can be valuable and informative.

14. The coach must make certain that his *players understand and follow the rules* and regulations of the game, with particular emphasis on those rules which have been designed to prevent serious injury, which should include an explanation to the players as to *why* certain rules have been designed to protect the player from injury.

15. Coaches should exert all their influence in the matter of *selection of* impartial and technically qualified *officials* who will properly enforce all the rules of the game at all times since the majority of rules are made to protect the players.

16. A good coach will, *with absolute authority, forbid playing tactics* which have been proven to increase the incidence of injuries to players. Four of the most serious ones are clipping, piling-on, spearing and grabbing the face bar.

Spearing is probably the most dangerous tactic that is used in football today and all knowledgeable people associated with the game of football are unanimously agreed that it *must be outlawed.* The pros long ago realized the danger inherent in the spearing maneuver and do not do it. In spite of this, some colleges persist in teaching spearing and it has even been taught to high school players! This is criminal! Why is spearing so dangerous?

First of all, the plastic encased helmet is a lethal weapon and with adequate force aimed at the mid-section of the opponent, can inflict serious and fatal damage, including damage to the heart, the spleen, the liver, and the kidneys.

Secondly, spearing has resulted in fatal head and neck injuries to players. If the head is directed into an opponent in an improper attitude resulting in acute flexion of the head on contact with the opponent, fracture-dislocation of the cervical spine can result with injury to the spinal cord, frequently resulting in paralysis and/or death. (See Chapter

5.) Few high school athletes have the neck muscles properly developed to the point of preventing acute flexion on sudden impact of the head with an almost immovable object—thus the head may acutely flex and the neck fractures, or the force of a head-on impact may cause fracture.

Why is *grabbing the face guard* so dangerous? Simply because this may result in an acute over-extension and/or rotation of the neck with serious injury to the cervical spine and/or neck muscles and ligaments. By outlawing such tactics, the life you save may be one of your players.

17. In the very near future, coaches will probably be asked to give consideration to *outlawing the use of the cross-body block,* since it is a major cause of knee injuries, mainly to the player receiving the block. In a recent report by Dr. Thomas R. Peterson* from the Section of Orthopaedic Surgery of the University of Michigan Hospital at Ann Arbor, it was emphasized that 54% of all knee injuries were caused by the cross-body block. A total of 189 knee injuries were studied over a 15-year period and included high school, college, and professional players.

Dr. Peterson emphasized that the cross-body block is used chiefly in the open field where considerable momentum can be developed and frequently it is inflicted on the defensive player from his "blind-side," when he is unaware of the impending block. He likened it to the thrust of a railroad tie against the side of the unprotected knee; in addition, he pointed out that injuries to the blocker who uses the cross-body block have at times been serious.

Dr. Peterson concluded that "As a result of this study I believe that football rules should be changed to eliminate the cross-body block. If other factors such as artificial turf and shoe variations should decrease the total number of knee injuries, there is reason to believe that the same percentage related to the cross-body block will persist."

18. The smart coach *never prolongs practice,* especially

---

*Journal of the American Medical Association, Jan. 19, 1970, p. 449.

contact practice, to the point of fatigue and exhaustion of his players. It has been a well-established fact for as many years as football has been played that the exhausted player is a prime candidate for an injury. Practice sessions lasting over 1½ hours are too long. Football at the high school level should be fun—and fun is winning! The tired team won't do well in practice and the tired team won't win the game.

If the scrimmage has been less than you as coach had desired, if less were accomplished than what you wished and, if the boys looked "terrible," part of it may be because the players are already tired. Obviously, this is *not* the time for heated emotions to rule your head and tell the manager to turn the lights on and "we'll stay here all night until we get it right." You'll get an unexpected injury or two every time, plus a bunch of tired, disappointed, and unhappy players. Thirty minutes of top effort scrimmage for a well-conditioned high school squad is sufficient—if they still look bad, everyone (including the coaching staff) will do better after a good night's rest.

19. The coach, of course, is responsible for establishing and enforcing a reasonable set of training rules for the players, including the usual recommendations regarding eating habits, proper and adequate sleep, attention to studies, avoidance of smoking and alcohol, suggestions concerning personal appearance and dress especially when playing out-of-town games.

20. If the coach does not have a *team physician* to work with, he should get one. Beg, borrow or steal—but by all means get a team physician to help in preventing and caring for the athletic injuries. If it is a small town, don't hesitate to ask the town physician—he will probably be more than glad to help. If it is a small town without any physician, find out if the closest city could furnish a physician at least for attendance at the regularly scheduled games. If necessary, call your County Medical Society and ask them for help in getting a team physician.

Chapter 7

CONDITIONING FOR THE ATHLETE

THERE is no question that the attainment of top physical performance is not possible without proper physical conditioning, which results in improved skill and coordination, and thus decreases injuries. Many contests are won in the last half by the team that shows the best physical condition. Most coaches have their own schedules of conditioning activities which usually include running, calisthenics and drills, stunts, and contests. For the best performance, conditioning should be a year-round program, sometimes difficult to achieve by the high school athlete who is only moderately motivated.

PREVENTING EARLY SEASON INJURIES

The most important aspect of proper conditioning from the medical standpoint is in *preventing early season injuries*. Extensive studies on injuries in football players have shown that almost 50% of all injuries occur in the *first three weeks of practice*, and 41% of all injuries occurred during scrimmage. This certainly emphasizes the need for longer and better conditioning before the hard hitting starts.

Further interesting and enlightening statistics on injuries during games show that fewest injuries occur in the first and last quarters of play, most in the second and third quarters. Some of these third quarter injuries might be prevented by adequate warm-up before the start of the second half. The studies further showed that ends, tackles, guards, and halfbacks were most subject to injury, while quarterbacks, centers, fullbacks, linebackers, and safety men were the least susceptible. The following outline will be helpful in planning a conditioning schedule.

1. At the end of the school year in June, coaches should give their athletes an outline of what is expected in the way of summer conditioning. For college athletes this is usually more vigorous than for high school boys. Coaches should emphasize the importance of this summer program. Conditioning exercises designed to strengthen neck muscles should be stressed.

2. Group conditioning exercises and games during the summer are not prohibited in most high schools, providing no member of the coaching staff is supervising organized conditioning. Most high school boys get together on their own and carry out sound programs, especially when directed by the junior and senior athletes.

3. Ideally there should be 18 to 21 days of conditioning and practice before the first scheduled game at the high school level. Eighteen practice days should be the absolute minimum if the coach is to condition the player and prevent unnecessary injuries. An interesting study was done with high school athletes in Rochester, Minnesota in 1961, comparing the physical fitness of two groups of players at one high school. One group started training in late July and spent 90 minutes a day for 5 days a week doing sit-ups, push-ups, wind sprints, jogging, long-distance running and stair running. In late August this group joined the second, unconditioned, group for regular football practice. Phys-

ical fitness tests showed that the pre-conditioned athletes scored higher than the others during all of September and October. Beginning in November the scores of the non-preconditioned athletes gradually increased until they matched those of the other athletes. The football season was about over by this time!

4. The first 7 practice days for any football squad should be done in shorts and T-shirts, football shoes and mouth pieces (for breaking-in), with *no contact* allowed. This is the time to push the conditioning exercises, but *not* the time to show how hard the boys can hit. This is the time for the coaching staff to evaluate the relative fitness of the squad and to find out who is and who isn't ready for the things to come. At the high school level, the fat boy who neglected summer training or the skinny sophomore with the long, lean neck may be the one to single out for longer periods of conditioning and muscle training before allowing him to get into contact drills. You might save an injury or a life!

5. When contact training starts, during the second week, start slowly and progress with the boys that are ready and fit—sort your squad carefully for those boys who obviously are not ready although they may be eager. The eager-unfit boys usually get the early injuries. Common sense and good judgment can prevent many early season injuries. Avoid punt and kick-off plays simulating game conditions since they can be hazardous in producing early injuries.

6. In research done recently on strength loss due to various phases of conditioning, it was pointed out that in *un-conditioned subjects* there was about a 25% loss in strength recovery remaining for *40 minutes after exercising to fatigue* in the first 2 weeks of training. It was therefore concluded that a rest period or a period of non-contact drill would be advisable for 30 minutes *after exercising* before starting contact drill, thus helping to reduce the early season injuries. As the athlete attains better conditioning, the

rest period between conditioning exercises and contact drill could be shortened, perhaps to 15 minutes.

7. Be sensible about *contact drills* without skipping the proper techniques. You can lessen the force of impact considerably by shortening the running distance before contact, whether it be contact with another player or contact with training equipment. After all, you're not trying to find out how great an impact a player can sustain without breaking something—you're trying to teach him techniques.

8. Don't *scrimmage* your squad when they are physically exhausted from too prolonged a period of conditioning exercises. On the days scheduled for scrimmage, give them a short warm-up drill, a few minutes of rest, then scrimmage. Be alert about a boy who may look tired, dragged-out, or dull in pre-scrimmage warm-up—he may be coming down with an illness, may have been short on rest, or maybe just isn't physically up to participation in scrimmage that day. This is the player than can suffer a serious injury that could have been prevented. If you feel they still need more conditioning, give it to them *after* scrimmage, *not before*. They may end up exhausted, but they won't be injured.

9. Most coaches will have a fairly good idea of the *relative fitness* of the squad after 10 or 12 practice sessions. One good way to help you evaluate fitness is to keep weight records on each player. This job can be delegated to a student trainer who will make up the chart and see that each player weighs in and out each day. The coach and team physician should study this chart every few days to see what the trend is. It will afford valuable information about excessive weight loss on unusually hot and humid days. It will tell you whether the fat boys are trimming down and the lean ones gaining weight. It will tell you if the average boy is losing too much weight and along with it his effectiveness. He may need more calories or he may need to check with his physician as to the cause of weight loss. Incidentally, don't rely on the standard height-weight

charts for ideal weights of athletes, since most of them are made up for ideal weights of non-athletes and do not consider body build and muscular development.

10. The most accurate and sophisticated method of measuring physical fitness utilizes the motor-driven tread mill. The term "physical fitness" here really measures functional capacity in relationship to the pulse and blood pressure response to a measured amount of exercise. This does not necessarily relate to muscular development or muscular strength. Since most high schools and smaller colleges do not have tread mills and physiology laboratories to help them, a simpler test for measuring physical fitness utilizes a prescribed number of steps on a 20-inch step, done in a given number of minutes. The pulse count following this exercise measures physical fitness when compared with the chart standards. If a coach is interested in such testing, ask your team physician to set up a program and to help in supervising it.

11. Coaches must remember that in conditioning training (high school level), it is one of their main duties to teach boys the fundamentals of gymnastics, tumbling, and rolling with a blow. It is not enough to teach the players how to make a good tackle or throw a good block, they must be taught how to behave *when hit*. Obviously, this will help prevent many injuries.

CONTROVERSIAL CALISTHENICS

There are not many of these to be considered, but four are worth mentioning:

A. The deep-knee bend and "duck waddle" are out and should never be used. They may cause serious and disabling injury to the knee joints.

B. The heel to neck arch (bridging) from the supine position can cause injury to neck structure in the high school athlete and should be avoided. Resistant-type exercises are far preferable, having the boys pair-up and exercise the neck against hand resistance.

C. The conventional "sit-up" exercise can contribute to low back trouble if done with straight legs. If the knees are bent until they are 6 to 8 inches off the ground and if the *head leads the body* in the sit-up movement, the exercise is of value.

D. Isometric exercises can build strength but they do not lengthen muscle fiber or produce movement. Isometrics alone are not desirable as a method of increasing *total fitness* but can achieve some results if practiced twice a day for 15 seconds each time for each muscle group.

WATER AND SALT INTAKE DURING PRACTICE AND GAMES

The much antiquated idea that water should be withheld from athletes during workouts and games has absolutely no scientific foundation. Water depletion in an athlete is more serious than water depletion in a sedentary person and can well lead to heat fatigue and/or heat stroke. An athlete can easily sweat out a quart of water per hour in hot weather workouts. In a recent survey (1969) it was shown that 56% of *high school coaches surveyed still limited water and salt intake during practice and games!*

How much water does the sweating athlete need to replace his loss during physical activity? The most reliable information will come from knowing his weight loss, and thus the importance of keeping accurate weight charts on each player. The best rule for water replacement is a weight-for-weight replacement, that is, a pint of water for each pound lost. Since weight loss will be quite variable among the players, so will the amount of replacement water required.

Weight losses of 2 pounds or less during activity pose no real problem to the players' fluid and electrolyte balance and will be easily replaced with small amounts of water during rest periods and the remaining after workouts.

Weight losses between 2 and 5 pounds require adequate replacement with water, some prior to activity, moderate amounts during rest periods, and the remaining amount afterward.

Weight losses exceeding 5 pounds call for frequent replacement of water during activity as well as some water-loading prior to activity. In these players it is wise to have them drink a pint of water before suiting-up for practice, perhaps another pint after suiting-up but allowing 20 to 30 minutes before beginning strenuous activity. In addition, it will be necessary to drink about ½ pint every 30 minutes during activity.

Obviously it is impossible to know *before* the work-out just how much weight each player will lose. Thus it becomes difficult to apply the above formula without information regarding weight loss. To solve this problem, make a practice of checking weight loss occasionally *on the field* before and after 30 minutes of strenuous activity. Do this during the first few days of practice, when players are not fully acclimated and when temperatures may be unusually high. This is the time when the greatest sweat loss occurs and fluid replacement is so very important.

Ideally, weight loss after strenuous practice should be checked with the player in the nude, since the uniform will absorb some sweat which has not yet evaporated, and thus one could actually underestimate the true weight loss. This factor would be relatively minor when the uniform consists of shorts and T-shirts during the first week of practice. It is advisable to have the player remove the T-shirt and weigh him with only shorts on if done on the field. However, if weights are checked on the field with the players in full uniform, then a greater allowance must be made for unevaporated water (sweat) in the uniforms. Your student managers can do this without upsetting the routine and the information will be very valuable in determining the needed water and salt replacements.

If weight checks are not done, then it is best to give the players *almost* all the water they want, short of distending their stomachs. Be generous rather than frugal. Have them drink some water prior to workouts, some during rest periods, and whatever they desire afterward. The average player will seldom over-load to the point of discomfort and in some instances coaches have said they must *encourage* players to drink water!

Depletion of the body electrolytes occurs during physical activity, particularly in hot weather, and replacement must be adequate. When we speak of electrolytes we refer mainly to sodium, potassium, and chloride. Ordinary table salt and salt tablets are sodium chloride; potassium replacement is discussed further in this chapter.

It is important to remember that the healthy human body possesses marvelous adaptive mechanisms to protect the individual from large electrolyte losses under ordinary conditions of exercise accompanied by sweating. However, this adaptive mechanism may be subnormal before adequate acclimatization has occurred, a situation that is frequently encountered in the first few weeks of practice when the weather is unusually hot and marked sweating occurs. This is the time when you must give special instructions to your players regarding salt and water replacement.

First of all, always advise your players to salt their food heavily.

Secondly, for all players whose weight loss exceeds 1 pound per workout, salt tablets should be taken. Preferably salt tablets should be taken with meals or immediately following meals to avoid stomach irritation, which can result in cramps, nausea, and vomiting. However, some coaches prefer to distribute salt tablets to the players immediately following workouts, in which case it is probably best to use the coated type to minimize gastric irritation. *Never make the mistake of giving salt tablets before the player has adequately replaced his water loss!* Serious disturbances of the body's electrolyte balance could possibly occur if salt is given before adequate water replacement.

How many salt tablets are required per day? Early in the season, when temperatures may be unusually high and acclimatization has not taken place, the players will sweat more profusely, weight loss will be appreciable (in some instances 5 to 8 pounds), and more salt will be required for replacement. At this stage, two salt tablets (7½-grain or 500-milligram size) per pound of weight loss will be adequate for most players who are not yet fully acclimated. In general it is best to limit the total number of salt tablets to *not more than* 12 per day, even though a player may on occasion lose *more* than 6 pounds per workout. It is also recommended that the tablets be given in divided doses with meals.

In the case of the player who has done physical labor outdoors during the summer months or who has had several weeks of pre-season conditioning and work-outs, less salt will be required. For this individual, one 7½-grain salt tablet per pound of weight loss will probably be sufficient.

After the first 10 days of practice when the temperatures are apt to be more moderate and the players are more fully acclimated, less salt replacement is required and one 7½-grain tablet per 2 pounds of weight loss plus heavy salting of food at the table will probably be sufficient.

When weight loss from sweating becomes minimal or negligible, then most team physicians and trainers feel that salt tablets are no longer necessary unless the athlete particularly requests them.

Since the major portion of salt loss from the body of the working athlete occurs in the sweat, it is obvious that when sweating is less, less salt replacement is necessary. In some parts of our country where temperatures remain high through most of October, sweating will be greater and some salt replacement will be necessary for more than the first 10 to 14 days of practice.

However, from the studies that have been done on the actual salt content of sweat, it seems quite apparent that as the individual adapts and becomes acclimated to heat stress, the salt content of the sweat decreases appreciably and in some cases has been found to be almost nil. Thus, even though appreciable sweating may continue in the warmer climates throughout the football season, the actual salt loss in most players will be much less than during the first few weeks of practice. One tablet per 2 pounds of weight loss in this situation will probably be adequate. Further research on salt loss in athletes will eventually give us a clear picture of the exact replacement necessary.

Remember again that the salt tablets should be taken in conjunction with the recommended volumes of water.

In the past few years several "special formula" drinks have become commercially available and have been advertised as being particularly beneficial to the athlete for replacement of water and minerals. These solutions usually contain potassium and sugar in addition to salt (sodium chloride) and are pleasantly flavored. They are also expensive.

Studies done at the National Institute of Health and elsewhere have shown that *prolonged and excessive* sweating may produce some loss of potassium from the body, although not sufficient to give rise to any signs or symptoms of illness. Therefore, unless there is an exceptional exposure to *severe heat-stress*, it would appear that furnishing extra potassium in these "special formulas" is probably not necessary, although certainly not harmful. Much of the food eaten in the daily diet contains potassium and one could be almost certain of adequate replacement by eating some of the high-potassium-containing foods each day, such as orange juice, tomato juice, bananas, apricots, cantaloupe, dates, and raisins.

If the team physician feels that there is a real need for potassium replacement, the following formula will make an acceptable and fairly palatable replacement drink, especially if well iced:

To each gallon of water, add the following:

1. One level teaspoon of table salt (sodium chloride)
2. One effervescent wafer of K-Lyte (available at most drug stores) which contains potassium bicarbonate.

3. Three to four tablespoons of sugar.

4. Flavor with 4 ounces of lemon, lime or grapefruit juice or other concentrated flavoring agents such as Kool-Aid.

This makes a solution which supplies 25 milliequivalents of potassium and 25 to 30 milliequivalents of sodium chloride per gallon, and is relatively inexpensive.

It is again emphasized, however, that under ordinary circumstances of practice, most athletes will maintain normal electrolyte and water balance by replacing water frequently and generously (at least 1 pint per pound of weight loss) and using extra salt on their food, plus taking the necessary salt tablets with or following their meals if temperatures are unusually high and sweating is quite profuse. I am grateful to Dr. R. L. Westerman of the Human Health Research and Development Laboratories, Dow Chemical Co., for his suggestions and advice concerning water and electrolyte replacement.

HEAT STROKE AND HEAT EXHAUSTION

Each year a few athletes lose their lives because of heat stroke and heat exhaustion. *These deaths are all preventable* if you will remember and follow these rules:

A. Schedule workouts during cooler morning and evening hours in hot weather, (meaning mid-day temperature over 80°F., with high humidity). Most deaths from heat strokes occur in the first 3 days of practice.

B. The first 7 practice schedules in hot weather should be in white T-shirts and shorts. T-shirts and shorts should be loose and permeable to moisture to provide maximum cooling. Soggy wet T-shirts should be changed for dry ones. Under no circumstances should a player be allowed to work out in any type of rubberized or plastic-type suit. These prevent almost all body cooling and are *very hazardous*. Likewise, sweat shirts and pants cut down efficient body cooling.

C. Acclimatize the boys to hot weather activity by carefully graduated practice schedules. In hot weather a session of 15 minutes work-out followed by 10 minutes rest has proven to be about right; or 20 minutes work-out and 15 minutes rest. Increase work-out time daily by 5 to 10 minutes, maintaining rest period of 10 to 15 minutes.

D. Make certain there is always adequate water replacement as indicated in the prior discussion.

E. Instruct all players about the need for extra salt as in the prior discussion.

F. *The full football uniform can actually be a death trap.* The risk of suffering heat exhaustion or heat stroke is increased by 50 to 75% when the player wears the heat-trapping uniform. It not only increases the work load by about 15 pounds, thus increasing heat production but since it covers the body surfaces so well, it also blocks effective evaporative heat loss over at least one-half of the body surface. To maintain body temperatures at normal levels the average football player produces and air evaporates 1½ to 2 pints of sweat per hour. If it is impossible to evaporate this much sweat by virtue of a tight cover on 50% of the body surface, the body temperature will start to increase.

It is imperative not to start wearing full uniform for the first 7 days of practice but to utilize T-shirts and shorts as indicated earlier in this discussion. Then, when uniforms are donned, begin by utilizing only part of the uniform such as helmets and shoulder pads and a light-weight permeable cotton jersey with short sleeves, plus shorts. A few days later, football pants with pads could be substituted for the shorts. Increase rest time in shade for the first few days of full uniform practice.

A study done a few years ago on 9 deaths from heat stroke in high school and college players showed that *all 9 of them* were clothed in full football uniform, all were interior linemen, and 7 of the 9 were stricken during the *first 2 days of practice* (in full football uniform)! It also was noted that 5 of these players who died from heat stroke were *not permitted water during practice* but were required to take salt tablets!

G. Weigh all players before and after work-outs; attempt to keep weight loss under 3% of their normal weight per day by adequate replacement of water.

H. Remember that players are acclimatized to the temperature and humidity in which they are practicing. If the temperature and humidity suddenly raise by 10 or more degrees, you have to start over with the precautions outlined in paragraph C above.

I. Most deaths from heat stroke occur in the parts of the United States where both temperature and humidity are high. The risk is far less where humidity is generally low and body cooling by evaporation is adequate. However, this *does not* mean that the need for water and salt replacement is any less.

J. *Be Alert to Signs and Symptoms of Heat Illness.* Observe players carefully for any of the following signs and/or symptoms which may forewarn of impending heat fatigue, exhaustion, or stroke. Fat boys are a 75% greater risk for heat illness.

1. Unusual fatigue, inattention, lethargy.

2. Awkwardness, sluggishness, or unusually poor performance.

3. Dizziness, thumping headache, nausea and vomiting.

4. Weakness with profuse sweating usually indicates an impending state of shock due to salt and water depletion and this is *heat exhaustion.*

5. A hot and dry skin with player in or near collapse usually indicates *heat stroke,* which can be fatal. The sweating mechanism has ceased to function and the body temperature is rising rapidly.

K. *Emergency Treatment of Heat Exhaustion or Heat Stroke.*

1. *Exhaustion.* Move the player to a cool, shady spot with head level with body and give sips of dilute salt water and obtain medical care at once.

2. *Stroke.* Act at once and act fast! Cool the body as fast as you can. Get the victim into cool water or ice the body

and obtain medical care at once. During transportation to a hospital, cooling of the body can be increased by covering the nude body with a light cotton sheet which has been well soaked in ice water and have the attendant continuously spray the covering with ice water. Fanning the body is also helpful.

All deaths from heat stroke are preventable—don't let it happen to one of your players.

SUNBURN

Most athletes have usually experienced enough sun exposure during the summer months to acquire an adequate tan which will protect them from sunburn during the days of practice in T-shirts and shorts. However, there is an occasional player who has not acquired this tanned skin protection and may be suspect to sunburn of the legs if not properly protected. If you have such players, make certain they are provided with lightweight cotton pants for at least part of the time that work-outs are conducted on sunny or hazy days. A bad sunburn can incapacitate a player for a week or more.

Chapter 8

PROTECTIVE EQUIPMENT AND PERSONAL CLEANLINESS

THE coach and team physician together must emphasize to the school's administration that a prime requisite in protecting the athlete from injury is adequate and top quality protective equipment. If the school cannot afford the best of equipment, they should not be playing football. To buy inferior or bargain basement equipment is jeopardizing the life and limb of the player and can only be condemned. Unfortunately there are presently no specific standards established or required as to the *best* type of equipment for all players. It is hoped that in the near future the Committee on the Medical Aspects of Sports of the American Medical Association and the National Federation of State High School Athletic Associations will make recommendations as to the most suitable and acceptable protective equipment.

A few of the basic principles are worth while reviewing here:

1. All protective equipment must be carefully fitted to the individual.

2. Check all equipment frequently for defects and wear and tear.

3. Used equipment that is defective should never be passed on to the B squad or the Freshman squad—they need as good or better equipment than the Varsity.

4. The coach must insist that all protective equipment be worn at all appropriate times—both in practice and in games.

5. Even the best equipment will not prevent *all* injuries but it will lessen the severity of most injuries and will certainly prevent many.

HELMET AND FACE BAR

The modern football helmet is a well-engineered protective device which protects the skull and its contents by spreading an impact over as large a surface as possible. Research has shown that an impact of 425 pounds per square inch to the head can fracture the skull. Yet football players sometimes receive *momentary* head blows in the magnitude of 300 G's or 300 times their weight in pounds. The *duration* of this impact has a definite effect on the degree of injury. A good football helmet will spread this impact over about 20 square inches with a minimum amount being transferred to the skull. In order to afford this great protection, the helmet must be fitted properly. Coaches and trainers must fit the helmets individually to each player, explaining to the newcomers exactly why a proper fit is so important.

Two types of helmets are presently being used. The commonest and most widely used type at the present time is the suspension type—with inner canvas web suspension, a sponge-rubber type padding, and an outer plastic shell. The newest type is the so-called "air" helmet (Micro-Fit, Riddell) which to date has been received with enthusiasm and some evidence that it probably affords greater protection than the older suspension type. This helmet is lined with 12 inflatable air pads, conforming exactly to the shape of the head. These air pads are inflated at five points on the top strap, the degree of inflation determining the proper fit. In addition, the air pads contain pads of vinyl foam and a layer of expanded polyethylene foam beneath the vinyl foam to provide added shock absorption and further protection in case the air cell should leak or rupture. The helmet further contains 12 hydro-cells, filled with water and methyl alcohol, which are activated when the inflated air pads are compressed by a heavy blow. The fluid in the wet reservoir is forced into another dry reservoir through a metering device in the event of a heavy blow.

The cost of this type of helmet is not much more than the conventional type and the teams that have used it seem to be quite enthusiastic about the protection it affords. Warn your players not to panic in case they feel fluid running down their face or neck from the region of the head! This is due to a ruptured hydro-cell and not a ruptured head!

For the players that still use the suspension-type helmet, the following outline will help in assuring a proper fit.

1. Before fitting the helmet, check that the suspension strap is tied properly.

2. Fit the helmet when the player has his regular hair-cut, since if he has a full head of hair when fitted and then gets a crew-cut, the helmet will need refitting.

3. If the helmet fits, it should turn only slightly when the player holds his head straight forward. The helmet should come down to about one fingerbreadth above the eyebrow.

4. When the player presses down on the helmet, or snaps the chin strap, he should feel the top of his head against the padded crown. If all pressure is felt on the forehead, the helmet is too low and needs adjustment. The suspension should just slide on the forehead with no large gap between.

5. Check the suspension on the side of the head by putting your finger in the ear hole to make sure the suspension band is touching the side of the head. If it is not touching the side of the head, the helmet will tend to move down over the base of the nose.

6. Jaw pads should be the correct size so that they fit snugly and prevent the helmet from lateral rocking.

7. Chin straps should be adjusted to the tight position with equal tension on both sides.

The face bar offers maximum protection from both soft tissue injury and facial bone fractures. In addition, it has minimized dental injuries. The face bar has been criticized by some because it may impair vision and because it has been used by some tacklers as a "handy handle" to bring the runner down. Minor to severe neck injuries have been reported as a result of this practice, but most coaches and physicians agree that the protection offered by the face bar outweighs the slight chance of serious injury. Most face bars are either the "bird-cage" type worn by linemen or the double-bar type worn by ball handlers. A good face bar should not protrude outward more than 3 inches.

MOUTH PROTECTOR

Use of the mouth protector is mandatory in most high schools now and has resulted in almost complete disappearance of dental injuries. Most football players can show the big smile with a full set of front teeth since the face bar and mouth protector have been required on high school players. In addition to protecting the teeth, the mouth protector has helped to dissipate jaw blows that could result in fractures of the jaw, concussion, and contusions. It has also minimized tongue and lip lacerations. There is also evidence that it provides some protection against neck injuries.

A good mouth protector must be comfortable in place, must allow ease of speech and ease of breathing and should be tear resistant.

There are three types of mouth protectors available—the stock, the mouth-formed, and the custom-made.

The "stock" or "boxer" type comes in one size, supposedly to fit everyone, is made of rubber or plastic, fits poorly, affords minimum protection, and generally is not recommended. Since they are cheap, some high school coaches advise their boys to use them. Unfortunately, this is poor advice.

Mouth-formed types are superior to the stock type and are popular and satisfactory. The kit consists of a horseshoe-shaped outer shell of firm rubber or plastic and an inner liner which is fitted to the individual's teeth. There are basically three types currently available, using either a combination of heat and cold to soften, fit, and harden the liner or a chemical softener. The most popular and satisfactory type is the polyvinyl acetate type that is thermoplastic, inexpensive, and can be resoftened and refitted if it becomes distorted and loose. The kit costs around $1.50.

Although complete instructions for fitting the protector come with each kit, it is preferable that a dentist be present to supervise the individual fitting. The coach or team physician can arrange with the local dentists to provide this service and usually the entire squad can be fitted in one evening if several dentists are present.

The custom-made mouth protector is processed individually by the dentist and is undoubtedly the most satisfactory type from all standpoints. However, this is relatively expensive and many players have to forego this procedure and settle for the mouth-formed kit variety. Certainly any players with unusual anatomy of the mouth must have a custom-made protector. Some quarterbacks prefer them because of greater ease of speech.

The mouth protector must be washed after each use (in cold water if thermoplastic type), which can easily be done when taking the shower. It then should be dried and stored in a perforated plastic box. A suitable wooden cabinet with compartments for each plastic box bearing the players' names has proven to be the best way of storing the mouth protectors between use.

Many players will avoid wearing mouth protectors if they can get by with it, especially if it is their first experience. An alert coach will have a spot check every few days to make certain the boys follow the rules.

In view of the great protection that mouth protectors provide, it is astounding that all college players are not required to use them.

PADS

Shoulder Pads. In football, the shoulder girdle receives impact more often than any other part of the body, and hence the necessity for adequate protection. Present day shoulder pads, now made of plastics, do an excellent job of protecting the shoulder, neck, and upper arm providing they are *fitted properly* and maintained adequately. Three important points must be stressed in the proper fitting and wearing of shoulder pads in order to afford the maximum protection:

1. Fitting should be done so that the pads snug into the neck as closely as possible and both halves of the pads should meet in the mid-line. The shoulder cap must fit over the deltoid muscle and not hang down on the arm. The back extension strap must be tight enough to prevent slipping and/or rotation of the pad. If pads are poorly fitted and loosely laced, they will slip from side to side over the shoulder girdle and injuries will result.

2. Properly fitting pads in conjunction with properly fitted helmets will prevent the so-called "pinched-nerve" or lateral neck sprain that so often happens. If there is too much space between the inner edge of the pad and the neck, then when the head is forced laterally it can be pushed down into this space with a resultant pull or pressure on the cervical nerve roots causing the symptoms of pain, numbness and tingling from the neck to the hand. If, on the other hand, the pads fit close to the neck, then the cheek pad area on the helmet acts as a brake and prevents excess lateral flexion of the neck.

For some players who have unusually long and thin necks, an additional felt collar may be helpful in preventing lateral flexion injuries.

3. The jersey plays an important role in keeping the

shoulder pads in place if it fits skin-tight. In addition, long, tight sleeves will be helpful in keeping the pad in place and will also protect the arm and elbow. On the other hand the loose fitting jersey allows the shoulder pads to easily slip out of proper position.

Do not allow your high school players to wear the smaller "pro-type" pads. They do not offer adequate protection in blocking or tackling and further they do not fit snug enough around the neck.

Hip Pads. Every player should wear hip pads, preferably the girdle type for the backfield and the conventional type for linemen. Hip pads must be worn high (above the top of the trouser line) to protect the lower back as well as to protect the crest of the ilium from the so-called "hip-pointer" or contusion to the iliac crest.

Thigh Pads and Knee Pads. In order that thigh pads and knee pads stay in their proper protective position, it is extremely important that football pants fit properly and fit snugly. Thigh and knee pads are important in protecting the player from painful bruises and in addition serve to soften the force of impact to the head of an oncoming opponent.

Rib Pads and Back Pads. Players who have sustained injuries to the region of the ribs or back frequently like the protection afforded by pads over these areas. Other special pads can be designed to provide protection for previously injured areas.

Elbow Pads and Forearm Protection. With the advent of artificial turf playing fields, it has become apparent that a relatively minor but definite hazard will be that of skin abrasions or "floor burns" due to sliding on the artificial turf, especially when it is bone dry. Since most players and many coaches object to long-sleeved jerseys, it is apparent that elbow pads and some type of forearm covering will be necessary to prevent numerous skin abrasions, since many such abrasions become infected rather easily and could thus incapacitate a player temporarily.

SHOES

Shoes as well as socks must fit properly in order to prevent blisters and calluses. Cheap shoes rarely fit well, so buy the best.

Since knee injuries constitute a major hazard to football players, a great deal of study has been done regarding the effects of different types or combinations of cleats on the incidence of such knee injuries. It is felt that some knee injuries can be prevented if the player can avoid having the feet firmly and deeply implanted in the turf at the moment of impact. Thus the leg receiving the blow can move away from the impact rather than be in a fixed position. Dr. D. F. Hanley team physician for Bowdoin College in Brunswick, Maine has done some valuable studies on this problem. Since there is considerable question as to whether heel cleats serve any real purpose on the football shoe, it is felt that modification of heel cleats will help to prevent firm fixation of the foot in the turf and thus prevent some knee injuries. The following modifications are currently being tested:

1. Replace the heel cleats with short soccer-type cleats.

2. Replace the heel cleats with a plastic circular disc or oblong plastic bar. (Easily put on with two screws fitting into cleat posts)

3. Replace the heel cleats with a $7/8$-inch high rubber heel, although some problems have been encountered with making the heel stay on plus the expense involved in installation.

According to studies on knee injuries and types of shoes reported to date, it seems apparent that knee injuries can be significantly reduced when the usual heel cleats are modified by one of the above methods. In detailed studies reported by Dr. Hanley, it was shown that guards and tackles suffer the greatest number of knee injuries. Twice as many knee injuries occurred on defense as on offense.

It would seem appropriate that any player who has previously sustained a knee injury would certainly benefit from modified heel cleats and further that probably all guards and tackles would likewise benefit.

There is certainly sufficient evidence that the long conical cleat should be discarded in favor of a shorter cleat on both sole and heel of all football shoes.

Shoes for Use on Synthetic Turfs. Since the advent of play on synthetic turfs, it has become apparent that a different type of shoe is necessary in order to provide adequate and proper traction on this type of surface. Although the perfect shoe is not yet apparent, several types are currently being tried.

It has been advocated by manufacturers of synthetic turfs that the incidence of knee injuries would be drastically reduced on such turf since it is impossible to plant cleats deep enough to firmly fix the foot. Although it is too early to compare statistics on all knee injuries occurring on natural grass turf versus synthetic turf, a recent study of the Seattle metropolitan league high school players has been reported by Dr. Harry Kretzler, orthopedic surgeon and team physician for Shorecrest High School in Seattle. His two year study would indicate that the incidence of knee injuries has been almost identical whether playing on natural turf or synthetic.

Three types of shoes have been tried on synthetic turfs:

1. The so-called "ripple-sole" shoe which is cleatless but has cross channels to provide traction. Experience with this shoe proves it provides good traction when the runner is going straight forward but inadequate traction when changing direction or "cutting."

2. A cleated shoe made with molded synthetic rubber cleats of the short soccer-type (½ to ⅝ inch long). The cleats are more numerous than on the regular style football shoe and some of them are placed well toward the perimeter of the sole thus providing better traction when changing direction.

3. A lug sole shoe which provides good traction but is heavier than others.

From the experience to date it would seem that the shoe cleated as above with soccer-type cleats is preferable on the *dry* synthetic turf but not as satisfactory on the wet synthetic turf. Some players prefer an ordinary tennis shoe on the wet synthetic turf.

It is obvious from this short discussion that the problem of proper shoes for use on synthetic turfs is still not completely solved and further study will be required before any definite recommendations can be made.

ANKLE WRAPS

The ankle joint is most vulnerable to injury in athletes and probably more so in basketball than in football. For this reason it is recommended that all players in both sports wrap their ankles for practice as well as games. This is best done utilizing a 2½-inch nonelastic wrap (woven cotton webbing), approximately 8 feet long. This is inexpensive and has proven to cut down the incidence of ankle injuries by 75%.

Wrapping is done either over or under the athletic socks and most coaches and trainers utilize a type of wrapping that has several turns over the heel, variously known as the Louisiana-style wrap or over-heel wrap. The players can be taught to do this themselves with a few demonstrations and then can either pair up or do it individually. These wraps should be washed at least weekly.

Adhesive wrapping of previously injured ankles is usually done by coach or trainer and the duration and extent of such wrapping must be determined by the physician and/or trainer. It is not felt that routine adhesive wrapping in a player with normal ankles has any advantage over cloth wrapping.

PERSONAL CLEANLINESS

In addition to supervising the purchase, fitting and maintenance of adequate protective equipment, the coach and team physician must impress upon the players the need for cleanliness and sanitation in other items of personal equipment.

T-shirts, supporters, and socks are frequently required to be furnished as personal equipment by the high school athlete and washing of these items is most often the players own responsibility. It is important from the standpoint of skin diseases, boils, and superficial skin infections, that such underclothing be kept clean and be changed or washed every day. A washer and dryer as part of the dressing room equipment are a good investment. Never allow the players to borrow the other fellow's equipment, since many skin disorders are contagious, including some potentially serious ones such as impetigo.

In addition, general cleanliness and order in the locker room is a must and the student trainer and aides should be responsible for this. The floors should be kept clean and the lockers not cluttered with left-over lunch, soft drink bottles, and other hazards to health and body.

Footbaths of various antiseptic solutions in an effort to prevent "athlete's foot" usually will contribute to the problem rather than relieve it and are *worthless*. Teach the player to dry his feet carefully, especially between the toes, to change socks daily, and for those who perspire freely to use ordinary talcum powder before putting their socks on in the morning and after practice. Emphasize personal cleanliness to your players—if they have not learned it at home, they could learn it in the locker room.

Towels in the Locker Room and on the Playing Field. Each player should be furnished a clean towel each time he showers—do not allow interchange of towels, they can transmit infections. The common practice of having one towel passed around during time out for all players to use for wiping faces or blowing noses is a good way to spread all sorts of infections among players. Excretions from the nose and mouth can be easily passed from one to another. Obviously it's impractical to have the trainer or water boy run on the field with 11 different cloth towels, so use paper towels of good absorbent quality.

Water for the Players. The common drinking cup is even more dangerous than the common towel. One player who may be incubating a respiratory infection, a sore throat, or even a contagious disease can pass his infection on to every other player through the use of a common drinking cup or jug or bottle. Avoid the use of these and use either a gallon or larger thermos jug with spigot and individual paper cups, or an atomizer-type of container which sprays the water directly into the player's mouth. These items may cost more, but in the end it will cost much less in terms of time lost from illness.

Remember the health practices you carry out on the playing field are observed by thousands of spectators (including parents) and it pays to always set the best example.

Chapter 9

FOOD—VITAMINS—OXYGEN—
DRUGS—SMOKING

SINCE so many misconceptions, fallacies, and unscientific beliefs exist regarding diets, drugs, and vitamins for the athlete, this chapter will emphasize the salient points that are important for the coaching staff and athletes to understand. Some athletes have the misconception that by eating some magic formula of special foods or special vitamins a "super-athlete" will emerge in due time. Unfortunately no such formula exists but certainly a properly balanced diet is vitally important to keep the athlete in good health.

GENERAL DAILY DIET

A good diet will furnish the body with carbohydrates, proteins, fats, minerals, roughage and vitamins. An athlete requires the same variety and balance of food as the non-athlete, to include the following:

1. *Bread-cereal group.* Four or more daily servings of

breads and cereals, preferably those that are enriched, restored or whole grain since they give considerable iron and B vitamins. This group furnishes mainly carbohydrates.

2. *Dairy foods.* Four or more glasses of milk daily and/or other foods made with milk, such as cheese, ice cream, or milk shakes. This group furnishes protein, fat and carbohydrate.

3. *Meat group.* Three or more servings daily of meat, poultry, fish, eggs, or cheese will supply most of the daily protein intake. Beans, peas, and peanut butter are alternatives, relatively high in protein. In addition, these foods (except cheese and fish) also furnish some iron and B vitamins.

4. *Vegetable-fruit group.* Five or more servings daily to include some green, leafy vegetables as well as a serving of a yellow vegetable such as carrots or sweet potato to help supply vitamin A. Most important, a citrus fruit or tomatoes, or citrus fruit juice or tomato juice should be included in the daily diet for their vitamin C content. Cantaloupe, strawberries, cabbage and potatoes are also good sources of vitamin C. Vegetables and fruits furnish mainly carbohydrates; some vegetables furnish moderate protein (dried peas and beans).

The discussion of proper diets for athletes frequently infers that probably most athletes eat a well-balanced nutritious diet at all times. I firmly believe that many high school athletes are deficient in some or many aspects of a proper diet and many studies in the teen-age groups have proven that there is a real need for education in proper dietary habits. Certainly in many families, no supervision of proper dietary intake or complete ignorance of what *is* a proper diet exists.

The college athlete who eats at a training table undoubtedly gets well-balanced and adequate diets during this period and at the same time learns what composes such a diet. However, consider the high school athlete from a home where perhaps both father and mother work and much of the diet consists of "snacks" put up by the athlete himself. He is probably a victim of malnutrition in one or more forms, although it may not be obvious from superficial examination. In some low-income families there may not be sufficient money to purchase adequate and proper foods. I believe it is vitally important that the coach assure that each boy understands what composes a good diet. It would be wise to give each boy a book or pamphlet which outlines the essentials of a good diet. Such pamphlets are available without charge from the local office of the National Dairy Council. Or contact: National Dairy Council, 111 N. Canal St., Chicago, Illinois 60606. This excellent booklet is titled *A Boy and His Physique*. In addition, the team physician should lecture to the squad about a proper diet and proper eating habits.

The following are some of the important points that should be emphasized:

1. Insist that your players eat a wholesome breakfast. Studies done on athletes have shown that this is an important meal in order to maintain peak performance. High school players frequently skip breakfast, either because of poor appetite at that time or insufficient time, usually the latter.

2. Three meals a day is the minimum for any athlete, and the growing high school athlete probably will want a mid-afternoon snack plus a bedtime snack to satisfy his needs for growth, development, and energy output.

3. Very high protein intake and protein supplements will not build super muscles or improve muscular strength and coordination. A liberal amount of protein is required, but not an excess.

4. Carbohydrates furnish an immediate source of calories and are important in the athlete's diet.

5. "Fad foods" have no place in the athlete's diet—nor do they impart any special substance to the diet that cannot

be furnished in a normal diet. Such foods would include yogurt, honey, protein pills, "energy pills," and others.

6. Milk is a good food for athletes and does not "cut wind" or impair athletic performance as some boys have been led to believe.

7. In preparing your athletes for the game, make use of the knowledge gained from important studies done on nutrition in athletes by Dr. Per-Olof Astrand, an eminent physiologist in Stockholm, Sweden.

Assuming a game is played on Saturday, it is customary for the coaches to curtail strenuous work-outs for about 48 hours before the game. Since during this 48 hours the muscles are recovering from the previous strenuous training, it would be wise to furnish a diet that is higher in carbohydrate and lower in protein to assure that the muscle and liver stores of glycogen (sugar) will be adequate to sustain the energy output needed during the game.

The following information is quoted from a recent article by Dr. Astrand*. "Protein is not a special fuel for working muscle cells. Fats and carbohydrates are. How much of each is used depends on the work performed. During mild exercise, fat is the prime fuel. As the exercise becomes more rigorous, carbohydrates become more important, until finally all muscle energy comes from this source. Diet greatly affects the relative participation of fat and carbohydrate in work metabolism. Consumption for several days of a carbohydrate-rich diet will improve capacity for prolonged exercise. Glycogen stores, which are strongly influenced by diet composition, are very important. The higher the glycogen content, the better the performance."

8. Maintain a weight chart for the squad and insist that each player weigh in and out for each practice session. A student trainer can be put in charge of this detail.

---

*"Something Old and Something New—Very New"—Per-Olof Astrand, M.D. Nutrition Today, June 1968, p. 9.

CALORIC REQUIREMENT

How many calories does the high school athlete require for adequate performance, to maintain ideal weight, and to provide for normal growth and development? Most foods furnish calories for energy; carbohydrates (sugars and starches) and proteins furnish 4 calories per gram, while fat furnishes 9 calories per gram. Caloric requirements depend upon the energy expended per day and if more calories are consumed than are used, the extra amount is stored as fat. On the other hand, if the diet supplies fewer calories than are used, body tissues are utilized to make up the difference and the individual loses weight.

In the high school athlete, the age, rate of growth, and actual body size affects the amount of calories required, but equally important is the physical activity that takes place daily. Obviously no two boys burn the same number of calories in physical activity, but we can be fairly accurate in predicting the number of calories needed per pound of weight in the *same age groups*.

The 15- to 18-year-old boys generally require about 25 calories per pound of body weight per day for normal daily activity. This would mean that the 150-pound boy requires about 3750 calories per day for normal activity. However, for the athlete who participates daily in a vigorous sport, it is generally agreed that he will probably need about 10% more calories for this physical output, which would mean that the 150-pound boy would consume around 4000 to 4500 calories per day. The 200-pound athlete will probably consume 5000 calories per day and utilize all of it. Keep in mind that these are approximate and will serve as a useful guideline, not as rigid rules.

To further the coaching staff's knowledge of what constitutes an average well-balanced and nutritious diet for the average 15- to 18-year-old high school athlete, the following page gives a sample diet of 4500 calories, including a bedtime snack. I am grateful to Mrs. Roberta Omans, Registered Dietitian, for setting up this diet

SAMPLE DIET OF APPROXIMATELY 4500 CALORIES

Breakfast:

    8 oz. glass orange juice or citrus fruits

    2 eggs

    3 slices bacon or ham

    1½ cups dry cereal or 1 cup cooked cereal

    2 - 8 oz. glasses whole milk (some for cereal)

    2 slices toast with butter or margarine

    Jam or jelly on toast if desired

Lunch:

    2 sandwiches (4 slices bread and 4 oz. meat, cheese, fish, or poultry)

    1 large apple or orange

    Butter or mayonnaise for sandwich

    4 cookies or 1 piece cake

    2 - 8 oz. glasses whole milk

Dinner:

    ½ lb. meat, fish or poultry

    Tossed green salad with dressing

    Buttered peas or other cooked vegetable

    Mashed potatoes and gravy

    2 Dinner rolls and butter

    2 - 8 oz. glasses whole milk

    Ice cream, pie or pudding

Bedtime Snack:

    1 sandwich (2 slices bread and 2 oz. meat, cheese, fish or poultry)

    Butter or mayonnaise

    Generous portion of fresh or canned fruit

    1 - 8 oz. glass whole milk

Approximate composition:

	%	Grams
Carbohydrate	40	421
Protein	17	200
Fat	43	215

PRE-GAME MEAL

1. Avoid excesses of protein such as the formerly accepted idea of steak and eggs for breakfast. Proteins are not the best source of fuel for the working muscles.

2. Feed mainly carbohydrates (sugar-containing foods) such as toast with honey, jelly or jam, cereals, peaches or pears in heavy syrup. Carbohydrates are 10% more efficient than proteins or fats in utilizing oxygen.

3. Give the pre-game meal 3 or more hours before the event so that the stomach is adequately emptied by game time.

4. For players with the "nervous stomach," individuals who may habitually vomit before a contest, or for those who feel "heavy in the stomach" at the start of the game, the use of a commercial liquid formula may avoid this trouble. Some of the better-known formulas are Nutrament (12½ oz. can supplies 400 calories); Metrecal (225 calories per can); Carnation Instant Breakfast (290 calories per glass when mixed with whole milk); and Meritene (270 calories per glass when mixed with whole milk). A recent study done by Mrs. Omans showed that Carnation Instant is the cheapest, costing .078 cents per calorie; Meritene next at .085 cents per calorie; Nutrament third at .13 cents per calorie.

Any of the above preparations may be given 2½ to 3 hours before the game. The advantage of a liquid pre-game meal is that it usually empties out of the stomach by game time and also provides calories needed for performance, thus an advantage in the athletes with the pre-game tension who might have stomach cramps, nausea, and vomiting during game time. It *does not* provide any greater source of energy or have any mysterious advantage over an ordinary high-carbohydrate pre-game meal, and certainly not all athletes require it, nor do some particularly like it.

In addition, liquid meals may be used as a daily supplement to regular meals to help underweight players gain weight. Powdered milk is an economical way of adding calories to the underweight players intake. Four tablespoons of powdered milk stirred into a glass of regular milk will add 56 calories—8 grams of carbohydrate and approximately 6 grams of protein.

HALF-TIME LIQUIDS

There is no agreement among authorities concerning half-time liquids. For most players plenty of cold water will satisfy them and they should drink *all they want*. If the weather is unusually hot, 6 to 8 ounces of the liquid formula given in Chapter 7 might be helpful.

For the athlete who "poops out" by half-time or feels unusual fatigue, it would be appropriate to give him a little carbohydrate boost with a fresh orange or orange juice, hot or cold tea with sugar added, or soft drinks.

CRASH DIETS AND DEHYDRATION TO PRODUCE WEIGHT LOSS

All physicians vigorously condemn the use of crash diets and dehydration to obtain a rapid weight loss in athletes, and particularly so in wrestlers. Weight loss by dehydration (sweating it out) can only lessen the athlete's immediate effectiveness and most of the lost fluid will be replaced in the following 48 hours by excessive water intake to replenish the badly needed body fluid.

The obese football player should have been trimming down during his summer work-outs but frequently he avoids this opportunity and turns out at a weight far in excess of his optimal for the most effective performance. In such cases it is prudent for the team physician or the personal physician to prescribe a reducing diet based on sound nutritional principles, which will allow a moderate but continuous daily weight loss until ideal weight is reached. The standard height-weight charts are designed for the non-athletic population and do not apply well to the heavily muscled athlete. The team physician should determine the ideal weight for the individual.

VITAMINS AND OXYGEN

Vitamins, when prescribed by a physician for a specific need, are valuable. There is really no evidence that an excess of vitamins will provide superior individual or team performance, nor will they prevent colds or similar minor illnesses. Many high school coaches and team physicians are aware of the fact that some players do not eat an adequate diet at home for various reasons. This situation could produce a border-line vitamin deficiency, occasionally enough to impair top physical performance. Certainly it is prudent to furnish these boys with a daily multi-vitamin supplement, which in most cases will be furnished by the school. These can be purchased in large lots through a pharmacist or wholesale drug company, making the cost fairly reasonable. The team physician should determine the type of vitamin to purchase and whether or not there exists the need for a multi-vitamin supplement.

No harm can be done by such vitamin supplements if one gives the type which provides the *daily* vitamin requirements and *avoids* the use of the "super-vitamin" which may furnish 5 to 10 times the daily requirement and is more costly.

Some coaches feel there is some psychological benefit to the players associated with furnishing them with vitamins.

Oxygen inhalation before or during a contest is probably not harmful and is of questionable physiological benefit, although perhaps of some psychological benefit. Oxgen cannot be stored so at best the inhaled oxygen can last only 2 or 3 minutes. If a player feels it helps him, certainly no harm can be done. Further scientific observations are needed before positive statements pro or con can be made.

DRUGS

Drugs or chemical compounds taken by athletes to enhance performance should neither be tolerated nor encouraged by coaches, trainers, or physicians. The International Amateur Athletic Federation has ruled that no agent which stimulates muscles and nerves, or paralyzes the sense of fatigue, or is habit-forming, should be used. The use of any drugs or dope in athletes has likewise been outlawed by the United States Olympic Association and The Amateur Athletic Union.

With our present problems concerning the relatively wide-spread use and abuse of potent and harmful drugs by some high school and college students, it becomes terribly important that all team physicians, coaches and trainers be exemplary in the field of athletics by condemning the use of any drugs by athletes except under the direct supervision of their physician.

Amphetamines. The amphetamines, commonly known as "pep pills," act to stimulate the central nervous system, lessen fatigue sensations, and constrict blood vessels. Common names of some are Benzedrine, Dexedrine, and Desoxyn. Some athletes call them "bennies."

Scientific studies of the amphetamines are not in agreement, but there is evidence that they may in some circumstances improve performance. However, in more complicated problem-solving situations there may be impairment of the individual's ability to solve a problem. In addition, there is the hazard of addiction and habituation. In excessive doses, the amphetamines can be very toxic and induce psychoses, hallucinations, and abnormal behavior.

A special committee of the American Medical Association, after exhaustive studies and investigation, concluded that "the use of amphetamines to improve athletic performance is inconsistent with the practice and ideals of sportsmanship and since their repeated use may be associated with harmful effects, the Committee strongly condemns the prescription of these drugs for this purpose by physicians, or their administration or use in athletics by coaches, trainers, or participants."

Androgenic-Anabolic Steroids. A relatively new group of drugs known as anabolic drugs has been under some discussion by coaches and trainers regarding their use in increasing muscle strength and promoting weight gain. These androgenic-anabolic steroids are closely related to the male sex hormone, testosterone, and are sometimes prescribed by physicians for undernourished and debilitated patients, frequently following major surgery and severe illnesses. These drugs have *absolutely no value* and offer no help to the healthy athlete and will not make him stronger in any way. More important still, they may manifest *serious but subtle side effects* which can be harmful to the health and body of the person taking them. These drugs can upset the hormonal balance in boys both before and after puberty and thus have an effect on growth, on normal testosterone secretion, on size of testicles (prolonged use can cause testicles to shrink) and on liver function.

Recently a carefully evaluated study done with athletes showed *no improvement* in strength, motor performance or work capacity in those who were given the drug compared with those who received no drug.

These drugs should not be given to healthy athletes of any age.

The Use of Oral Enzymes. Enzymes, both proteolytic and non-proteolytic have been prescribed by many team physicians in an effort to hasten healing and absorption of blood from a bruised and sprained area. Well-documented studies seem to show some decrease in healing time, while others show equivocal results.

Since there are almost no known serious side effects from the use of these preparations, the decision as to their use with a given individual should rest with the team physician.

Tranquilizers and Sedatives. The healthy, well-motivated, athlete certainly does not require the use of daytime tranquilizers or sedatives to calm his nerves the day before or the day of a contest. There is real evidence that such medication may result in ineffective performance with slowing of both physical and mental activity. A moderate amount of nervous tension is normal in many players prior to competition and this feeling usually disappears after the first play.

The player that is so "keyed-up" that he cannot sleep at all the night preceding a game probably will be helped with a mild, short-acting sedative properly prescribed by the team physician or family physician. There is no argument with the fact that 8 hours of sleep aided by a mild sedative is far preferable to no sleep simply because someone may have a "moral objection" to the use of any such sedatives. A cup of strong coffee with breakfast will neutralize any "hang-over" effect, if such occurs.

Analgesics (Pain-killers). The use of strong analgesics, by mouth or by injection, for the purpose of reducing or eliminating pain in order to get the "star" back into the game at once can only be strongly condemned. First of all, if the injury is so severe as to require codeine, morphine or comparable strong synthetic analgesics for relief, it is very likely that the injury is severe enough to keep the player out of the game until complete evaluation of the injury is done by the physician, which in most cases would include an x-ray film of the injured member.

Secondly, the effects of drugs in this class are such that they dull the reflexes and the mind while relieving pain, and the athlete returning to a game would be not only ineffective but more vulnerable to further injury to the same area or to other areas.

Novocaine Injections. I have no intention of discussing in detail the merits or the hazards of the practice of injecting novocaine or a comparable local anesthetic into painful and injured areas in an effort to return the player to the contest at once. This practice is carried out by some physicians and by some trainers under the advice of the team physician. Most high school team physicians and coaches properly feel that such a practice has no place at the high school level and can well produce further injury.

There is no doubt that the injections of a local anesthetic into a painful area will dull the pain. However, there are many times when even an orthopedic surgeon cannot be sure from physical examination of the injury, whether or not the player has sustained a fracture and/or severe ligament injury. In such cases x-ray films are mandatory before treatment can be undertaken. The treatment of a mild sprain or a bruise is quite different than the treatment of a fracture, or ligament tear. Each year there are cases where a player has received an injection of a local anesthetic during the game, returned to play, then later was found to have a fracture. Everyone agrees that returning to play with an untreated fracture is not the best medical treatment for the player!

It must be concluded that injection of a local anesthetic into an injured extremity is not currently accepted as good practice. It should not be done.

SMOKING

For the coach who wants to put a little scientific evidence behind his rules against smoking, the following points might prove helpful:

1. The young athlete who wants to achieve top performance had best never start to smoke—it is a stubborn habit to break.

2. Carbon monoxide may be absorbed when smoking, thus reducing temporarily the oxygen-carrying capacity of the blood.

3. Smoking can produce digestive disturbances and dull the appetite.

4. Smoking can lead to nervous irritability, restlessness, and loss of sleep.

5. The absorption of nicotine from smoke can cause a constricting effect on blood vessels and contribute to the development of heart and circulatory disorders.

6. Smoke irritates the mucous membranes of the throat and lungs and in due time can lead to serious and chronic disorders of these organs.

7. There is definite statistical evidence that cancer of the lung is many times more frequent in heavy cigarette smokers. This point alone should discourage all of us from smoking cigarettes!

8. Smoking has *never* contributed in any way to athletic fitness.

Ideally your team physician should spend 30 minutes with your squad on a more-detailed discussion of these points.

Chapter 10

PSYCHOLOGICAL FACTORS IN THE PREVENTION OF FOOTBALL INJURIES

IT is neither my intent nor capability to write a detailed chapter concerning the psychological factors involved in the prevention of football injuries. However, since a great deal of interesting and valuable study is currently in progress in this area, it seems worthwhile to introduce the reader to some of the factors which may be of value.

There is certainly much truth in the oft-repeated statement that many football games are either won or lost as a result of what the head coach said to the players either before the start of the game or during half-time. Every year we see several "under-dog" teams upset the favorite and realize that this great motivation came about through the utterings of an inspired coach. Knute Rockne was probably the greatest example of a fine coach whose knowledge of psychology equaled his coaching skill.

All coaches should be good students of psychology and know how to apply it. Unfortunately, this goal is achieved by very few and then only after many years of observation and experience. I believe that all football coaches would be more successful if they showed a greater interest in and understanding of some of the emotional conflicts apparent in certain players. There is a great need for more communication between the psychologists who are studying the problems and the coaches. There is much to be learned that will probably result in better performance by the players. There is also much to be learned that will prove valuable in injury prevention. Coaches are like all other people in that they have preferences for certain types of individuals. The coach has pre-formed ideas of what characteristics and qualities define the "good athlete." Some coaches may tend to reject an otherwise fine athlete simply because he displays certain personality traits that irritate or "bug" the coach. This rejection may well create a severe emotional conflict in the player which in turn may contribute to an injury.

A recent book entitled *Problem Athletes and How to Handle Them* by Ogilvie and Tutko (see Appendix) devotes a chapter to the coach and his personality and is worthwhile reading.

There is no question that psychological factors contribute to *some* injuries. Athletes undergo the same emotional conflicts that affect all of us in everyday living. In addition, however, certain conflicts become apparent in relationship to competitive sports and these involve not only the desires of the athlete himself, but the demands of others—coaches, parents, teammates, teachers, the student body, and spectators.

All successful athletes must be aggressive whether in team sports or individual sports in order to give their best in an effort to win. However, many athletes have developed conflicts concerning aggression dating from infancy and childhood, and some of these conflicts may be solved when an athlete sustains an injury.

The injury-prone athlete has been studied rather extensively by psychologists in an attempt to learn more about the emotional make-up of these individuals and what, if anything, can be done to help them avoid injuries, which frequently seem to plague some of them all through their athletic careers. Some injury-prone athletes never seem to learn from experience and thus are incapable of learning how to avoid injuries. Some may display a reckless as well as fearless attitude in practice and games, only to end up on the injured list time and again.

The psychologists tell us that one of the main reasons such an athlete continues to sustain injuries is that he *may want to be injured*. By being injured he thus can attain certain psychological needs that are otherwise impossible. By being injured, the player avoids competition. He wants to avoid competition because he feels inferior compared to his opponents and thus can avoid the threat of being a loser by not even being a contender. Certain other psychological benefits seem to be derived by some players who sustain frequent injuries, the psychologists say, which would include remaining as a member of the team without putting in the time and effort in practice; a feeling that the team owes him something for his great sacrifice; and of course much sympathy and attention from others. The injury-prone athlete is discussed in detail in the book referred to above.

How can the coach and team physician recognize the boy who might be subject to injury because of unrecognized emotional factors? There are a few definite situations which might predict injury potential.

1. A marked disproportion between a boy's athletic ability and his willingness to be aggressive may exist. This includes either a boy who has great aggressiveness but not a matching ability or the boy who has the ability but lacks aggressiveness.

2. A father-son conflict frequently forces a boy into sports for which he is neither physically nor mentally prepared or capable. On the other hand, the boy who becomes

more capable and aggressive than his athletically successful father, may face emotional conflicts.

3. The over-fearful or timid athlete, who slows down or lets-up at the crucial time for fear of sustaining an injury, is most frequently a prime candidate for injury.

4. An occasional athlete may try to conceal his injury, hoping to return to action sooner. A more serious injury could result or the original injury could be aggravated. This may be construed as a conflicted expression of aggression if one can prove that perhaps the athlete is seeking injury. In most cases it is probably an expression of mental toughness and a real desire to be part of the action.

5. An occasional athlete will exaggerate his injuries and demand more than the average attention and sympathy for a relatively minor injury. Since this may be a manifestation of an underlying fear, this boy should probably not be playing in a contact sport.

It seems entirely possible that through more extensive personality studies in athletes, one may be able to predict what particular traits are more apt to be associated with repeated injuries. One such study is being actively pursued by Bruce Ogilvie, Ph.D, and his associates, T. A. Tutko, Ph.D, and Lelean Lyon, M.A., in the Department of Psychology at San Jose State College. These men have designed an Athletic Personality Inventory (API) which is a paper-and-pencil test designed specifically to measure those traits which are related to high athletic achievement. The API gives measurements on 12 personality dimensions; desire, self-confidence, aggressiveness, coachability, determination, emotionality, conscience development, trust, response to pressure, guilt-proneness, leadership, and mental toughness. If from studies such as these a pattern of personality traits evolves that would predict the injury-prone athlete, then proper steps could be taken to avoid such injuries.

How does the coach and team physician handle injury-prone individuals in an effort to prevent injuries? Careful

counseling by the coach and team physician, may be helpful and all that is necessary. However, more serious problems should have counseling with a psychologist or psychi-
atrist who is experienced in athletic behavior and familiar
with the problems. In many instances it is prudent to suggest to the boy some other athletic endeavor where the
chances of serious injury would be minimal.

Chapter 11

TACKLE FOOTBALL IN
JUNIOR HIGH SCHOOL

EACH year more boys in junior high school are participating in tackle football either under sponsorship of the school administration, local sports-minded businessmen, or sometimes under national sponsorship. The Pop Warner League in football, Little League baseball, and Pee-Wee Hockey are some of the more popular sports.

Not all physicians and administrators are in agreement as to whether this is good or bad. As experience accumulates and records are reviewed, the general conclusion has been that the adequately administered programs are quite satisfactory. The percentage of injuries is less than anticipated, and the overall benefits seem to outweigh the risks. It seems quite obvious that boys of all ages seek outlets for their energies; that from a very early age competition is a way of life; and that in spite of some objections which may be well substantiated, the popularity of these competitive sports is going to increase instead of decrease. Statistics on injuries in football show that about one-fourth of the injuries occur in *unsupervised* sand-lot play. It seems obvious that *supervised* competitive athletics in this age group will certainly result in *fewer* injuries.

In 1958-59, the entire question was given considerable study by the Committee on the Medical Aspects of Sports of the American Medical Association and on February 1, 1959, the following report was adopted. "Inquiries concerning the advisability of conducting tackle football programs in junior high schools have recently been referred to the Committee on the Medical Aspects of Sports of the American Medical Association. The group involved would be youths in grades 7-9 inclusive, ranging in age from approximately 12-15 years. After carefully considering the various aspects of this problem, the Committee has issued the following statement:

"Whether junior high school boys should participate in tackle football has been a matter of considerable controversy with medical opinion ranged on both sides of the issue. The arguments advanced in support of each viewpoint are myriad but, in the opinion of the Committee, actual evidence is fragmentary and conflicting. Also, the Committee recognizes there are many educational factors to be considered.

"Because of the problems outlined above, the Committee feels that the decision as to what level to begin programs of contact sports will have to be made largely on a local basis. However, the Committee submits the following suggestions to local authorities considering the matter:

"A. With consideration for the health and fitness of *all children and youth*, local groups should make certain that physical education and athletic programs provide:

"1. A daily period of physical education for all boys and girls that includes a wide variety of activities and emphasizes careful instruction adapted to individual needs.

"2. Opportunity for all boys and girls to participate in an

informal play and intramural program that includes a number of team games as well as appropriate individual and dual sports.

"B. Having provided the above basic program, some communities may find it possible to offer certain specialized sports experiences; however, strenuous contact sports such as tackle football should be considered only when the following conditions for play can definitely be assured:

"1. A medical examination including a thorough review of health history before and as needed during the season.

"2. Careful matching of players by age-height-weight formula or other equitable basis.

"3. The best obtainable equipment for play, properly fitted to each player and with practical adaptations such as the use of tennis shoes.

"4. A faculty member (coach) in charge who understands child growth and development, as well as first aid, conditioning, and the sport concerned.

"5. A physician present at all contests and readily available during practice sessions.

"6. Officials thoroughly conversant with the limitations of young players as well as the rules of the game.

"7. Playing fields which meet standard requirements for size of area, playing surfaces and facilities for safety.

"8. Written agreement as to responsibility for injury incurred in athletics made known to all participants and their parents.

"C. In addition to assuring proper conditions for participation, a number of basic policies for play are required. It is essential that these include provision that:

"1. No games will be played until players are well-drilled in fundamentals and have had a minimum of two weeks of physical conditioning.

"2. The length of periods and the duration of the season will be appropriately modified in terms of the age of players.

"3. Suitable adaptations in equipment for safety and practicality such as the use of tennis shoes for younger age groups will be made.

"4. A player who has been ill or injured will be readmitted to participation only upon the written recommendation of a physician.

"5. Upon return to play, a participant who has been ill or injured will be carefully observed and referred to a physician if there is any doubt of his condition.

"6. When an injury occurs during the course of a contest, the physician in attendance will determine the athlete's ability to continue play.

"7. During practice sessions, in potentially serious injury, particularly to head, neck or spine, the injured player will be removed from play, placed at rest, and given the immediate attention of a physician.

"8. Emphasis will be placed on skillful performance, maximum participation, healthful play, and good sportsmanship rather than championship schedules and all-star teams.

"9. On all matters of procedure and practice not covered by these policies, the first consideration will be the health and welfare of players."

In Spokane, Washington, a group of dedicated business and professional men have sponsored a Junior Tackle Football program since 1966. Everyone connected with the program including parents, players, coaches, and team physicians, feels that it has been and will continue to be valuable. High school coaches have been particularly impressed with the improved ability and attitudes of the incoming freshmen who have previously participated in the junior program. In addition, it has given the players themselves an opportunity to evaluate their own desires as to whether or not they *really* want to be a football player in high school. They thus eliminate themselves by finding the sport not to their liking or their particular ability and perhaps switch to a different sport after entering high school.

We have insisted upon close supervision as well as careful selection of coaches, careful matching of players by age and size, physicians in attendance at all games, and a minimum of emphasis on championship contests. All players wear tennis shoes—no cleated shoes of any type allowed at any time—thus reducing cleat injuries. All players wear good equipment—the best that can be bought—including mouth guards for all players. All players on every squad, usually 25, *play equal time in every game* regardless of their ability. Practice time is carefully limited so as not to interfere with school work, meal times, and rest time. The emphasis is on *learning* the game rather than winning the game, but let's face it—they all want to win!

The program is run much like the high school programs from the standpoint of taking all possible steps to *prevent* injuries. There have been an average of five fractures per season—mainly fingers, arms, and clavicles, with about 400 boys participating, so the incidence is low. No serious or fatal injuries have occurred. No knee injuries have occurred.

If your community or school administration is considering such a program, it would be well to secure detailed information from organizations that have carried on such programs.

APPENDIX

American Medical Association Publications

(Published under the Auspices of the Committee on the Medical Aspects of Sports Division of Environmental Medicine).

1. Tips on Athletic Training—A series of booklets numbered I through XI. Available for 30 cents each in single copies from the American Medical Association, 535 N. Dearborn St., Chicago, Ill. 60610.

2. A Guide for Medical Evaluation of Candidates for School Sports. (1968) Available from American Medical Association for 25 cents each.

3. Standard Nomenclature of Athletic Injuries. (1966) Available from American Medical Association for $1.50 per copy.

4. First Aid Chart for Athletic Injuries. (Prepared by the AMA Committee on the Medical Aspects of Sports in cooperation with the National Athletic Trainers Association and the National Federation of State High School Athletic Associations.) Available in 10½" x 15½" Paper Edition for 30 cents each or 11" x 16" Plastic Laminated for $3.00 each from the American Medical Association.

5. Proceedings of the National Conferences on the Medical Aspects of Sports. Booklets containing the papers given at each annual National Conference from 1959 through 1966. Available at most Medical Libraries.

Medical Texts on Sports Injuries

1. Armstrong, J. R., and Tucker, W. E. (eds.): *Injury In Sport*, Springfield, Charles C Thomas, 1964.

2. Ferguson, A. B., and Bender, J. A.: *ABC's of Athletic Injuries and Conditioning*, Baltimore, The Williams & Wilkins Co., 1964.

3. Hirata, Isao, Jr.: *The Doctor and The Athlete*, Philadelphia, J. B. Lippincott Co., 1968.

4. O'Donoghue, D. H.: *Treatment of Injuries to Athletes, 2nd Ed.*, Philadelphia, W. B. Saunders Co., 1970.

5. Ogilvie, Bruce C., and Tutko, Thomas A.: *Problem Athletes and How to Handle Them*, Los Altos, California, Tafnews Press, 1966.

6. Novich, M. and Taylor, H.: *Training and Conditioning of Athletes*, Philadelphia, Lea & Febiger, 1970.

7. Ryan, A. J.: *Medical Care of the Athlete.* New York, McGraw-Hill Book Co., 1962.

8. Sills, F. D., Morehouse, L. E., and DeLorme, T. L. (eds.): *Weight Training in Sports and Physical Education*, Washington, D.C., American Association for Health, Physical Education, and Recreation, 1962.

9. Thorndike, A.: *Athletic Injuries—Prevention, Diagnosis and Treatment, 5th Ed.*, Philadelphia, Lea & Febiger, 1962.

10. Trickett, Paul C.: *Prevention and Treatment of Athletic Injuries*, New York, Appleton-Century-Crofts, 1965.

11. Williams, J. G. P.: *Sports Medicine*, Baltimore, The Williams & Wilkins Co., 1962.

INDEX